MRCP (Paed
Part 1 MCQs

S. Hannam, G.F. Fox and M.J. Marsh

MRCP (Paediatrics): Part 1 MCQs

Dr Simon Hannam

Senior Registrar in Paediatrics,
Department of Child Health,
King's College Hospital,
London, UK

Dr Grenville F. Fox

Fellow in Neonatology
Department of Paediatrics,
Hospital for Sick Children,
Toronto, Canada

Dr Michael J. Marsh

Consultant in Paediatric Intensive Care
Caleb Ward,
Guy's Hospital,
London, UK

W.B. Saunders Company Ltd
London • Philadelphia • Toronto • Sydney • Tokyo

W.B. Saunders   24–28 Oval Road
Company Ltd   London NW1 7DX, UK

The Curtis Center
Independence Square West
Philadelphia, PA 19106-3399, USA

Harcourt Brace & Company
55 Horner Avenue
Toronto, Ontario M8Z 4X6, Canada

Harcourt Brace & Company, Australia
30–52 Smidmore Street
Marrickville, NSW 2204, Australia

Harcourt Brace & Company, Japan
Ichibancho Central Building,
22-1 Ichibancho
Chiyoda-ku, Tokyo 102, Japan

A catalogue record for this book is available from the British Library

ISBN 0–7020–1875–9

Typeset by LaserScript, Mitcham, Surrey
Printed and bound in Great Britain by WBC, Bridgend, Mid Glamorgan

Contents

Preface

This book is written primarily for candidates studying for the Paediatric Part 1 examination of the Membership of the Royal College of Physicians of the United Kingdom (MRCP). It may also be useful for the preparations of candidates in other paediatric postgraduate examinations and medical students.

This branch of the MRCP examination has only recently been introduced and is clearly still in the process of evolution. The Part 1 examination is designed to test knowledge of basic medical science that has relevance to the practise of clinical paediatrics, in addition to a basic knowledge of important paediatric conditions. The examination is still in the form of a multiple choice question (MCQ) with true and false as the options. In preparation for the examinations we recommend that use is made of the many existing 'adult' based books that centre on many of the principals of basic medical science that you need to understand in order to pass the examination.

This book has been divided into five papers with a mix of questions that are similar in nature to the questions appearing in the examination. This format has been followed to simulate exam conditions in order to prepare for the examination in the most effective way. The PC disk provided in the book offers you the opportunity to study subject areas as well as perform an examination in a strictly timed manner – the computer times you and stops you from cheating!

This book contains 300 questions with the correct answers and explanatory notes. These notes are designed to inform you about the subject area but are by no means exhaustive. We recommend that as you find areas where your knowledge is deficient you make notes and refer to detailed texts to clarify the problem. This book will hopefully help you take the first step into a career in Paediatrics.

S.H.
G.F.F.
M.J.M.

How to Answer Multiple Choice Questions in the Paediatric Part 1 MRCP Examination

The Part 1 MRCP examination is a single paper containing sixty true or false multiple choice questions (MCQ) with each of the sixty questions having five parts. The time allowed for the examination is two hours. The marking system awards one mark (+1) for each item correctly answered (i.e. a true statement indicated as true or a false statement indicated as false). A negative marking system is in operation and for each item incorrectly answered (i.e. a true statement indicated as false or a false statement indicated as true) one mark is deducted (–1). If an item is not answered (Do not know) no mark (0) is awarded. The following guidelines should assist you in answering the questions correctly.

Read Questions Carefully

For each question it is important that you read the question carefully and ensure that you understand it before attempting the answer. It is best to return to the 'stem' question or statement when you consider each of the five parts and each item considered independently of the other statements. In view of the negative marking system you can not afford to make careless mistakes with any answers. In the two hours allotted you have to read, understand and consider answering 300 items and though it is important to plan your time carefully to avoid running out of time before all questions have been considered, it is easy to rush in and misread questions. Common mistakes include misreading words prefixed with 'hypo-' and 'hyper-'. Please read each and every word in the stem question and each part with care.

Do Not Read Between the Lines

Many exam candidates think that the questions have catches or
hidden meanings. Read and accept the questions at face value,
reading each carefully to avoid foolish mistakes. The exam is
designed to test your factual knowledge and questions have been
selected by the exam board to be free of ambiguities.

How Many Questions Should You Answer? To Guess or Not To Guess

Once you have read each item, it is likely that your initial response
will fall into one of three categories.

First, you are sure of the answer and have no doubt about the
correct response (whether true or false) in this case you should go
ahead and answer the question.

Second, there are those items about which you are uncertain
about the answer but there is a familiar 'ring' about the question. In
this case you may not immediately know the answer, but with some
careful thought and reasoning you may be able to work out the
answer from first principles. In this case it is more likely that your
answer is correct, and we would advise you to be bold and answer the
question accordingly (whether true or false).

Thirdly, you are maybe totally ignorant of the subject or
completely unsure of the answer. In view of the negative marking
system you should not guess blindly and therefore you are best
advised to answer 'Do not know'.

Plan carefully and Organize Your Time

With sixty questions in the two hours you have two minutes per
question or 24 seconds for each of the individual 300 items. This is
plenty of time since the items you are sure about only take a few
seconds to read and answer. This gives you the additional time that
you require to consider the questions using first principles before
giving your answers. You can either answer all the questions that you
are sure about by first marking your answers on the exam paper
immediately and then return to the others that you are uncertain
about. Alternatively you can mark your answers to all the questions
on the exam paper as you go through the first time keeping a careful
eye on the clock in order to avoid running out of time before

completion of the entire paper. *Remember that your first thought is likely to be the correct answer.*

Fill in the Answer Sheet Correctly

You must avoid making an error by recording an answer in the incorrect place since this may lead to a systematic error. If you answer question 1 in the place of question 2, all the following questions will be wrong and even if you discover this before the end of the examination it is difficult to correct and not panic.

Fill in the Answer Sheet Correctly

Paper 1

1. **The following occur in childhood asthma:**
   A. cough as the predominant symptom.
   B. stridor.
   C. increased airways resistance.
   D. decreased lung compliance.
   E. decreased functional residual capacity.

2. **Oral rehydration therapy:**
   A. works by passive absorption of glucose.
   B. is effective in 50% of moderately dehydrated infants.
   C. should not be used in hypernatraemic dehydration.
   D. contains 5 mmol/l of potassium.
   E. can be made up safely at home using salt and sugar.

3. **Recognised causes of hypertension in childhood include:**
   A. chronic glomerulonephritis.
   B. renal vein thrombosis.
   C. neuroblastoma.
   D. coarctation of the aorta.
   E. congenital adrenal hyperplasia.

4. **A 6-week-old male infant is admitted to hospital with 10–15% dehydration. The serum sodium is 160 mmol/l and the serum potassium is 3.3 mmol/l:**
   A. congenital adrenal hyperplasia is a likely diagnosis.
   B. loss of skin turgor is likely to be present.
   C. the dehydration should be corrected over the next 2–4 hours.
   D. bloody diarrhoea suggests a bacterial cause.
   E. initial fluid replacement should be with 0.45% saline.

1. **AC**
   Persistent cough, especially at night, is often a presenting feature of childhood asthma. Stridor is a feature of upper airways obstruction and therefore does not occur in asthma. Increased airways resistance occurs in asthma. This leads to air trapping and increased Functional Residual Capacity (FRC). Compliance is normal.

2. **All False**
   Oral rehydration therapy works as glucose is actively absorbed across the lumen of the intestine in a cotransport system with sodium. It is effective in up to 90% of infants in the UK with moderate dehydration. Oral rehydration therapy is the treatment of choice for hypernatraemic dehydration as there is a more gradual correction of electrolyte imbalances than using intravenous therapy. All oral rehydration solutions contain potassium concentrations of 20 mmol/l. Solutions made up using home ingredients should be discouraged because of the possibilities of making hypertonic solutions.

3. **ABCDE**
   Investigation of hypertension in childhood must always include examination of the urine for albumin, red cells and casts. This will exclude chronic glomerulonephritis. In addition urine should be collected to detect the presence (or absence) of catecholamines. Hypertension can be seen in congenital adrenal hyperplasia in both 11-beta-hydroxylase and 17-hydroxylase deficiencies.

4. **DE**
   The most likely cause of hypernatraemic dehydration in infants and children is infective diarrhoea. This is likely to be bacterial if the stool contains blood. The skin may have a doughy consistency in hypernatraemic dehydration. Rapid correction of the increased serum osmolarity results in intracellular fluid accumulation, which may lead to cerebral oedema. This can be avoided by slowly correcting the fluid depletion (over 24–48 hours) and ensuring that the serum sodium is lowered at a rate of no greater than 10 mmol/l/24 hours.

5. **The following are recognized risk factors for neonatal group B streptococcus (GBS) infection:**
   A. preterm labour.
   B. prolonged rupture of membranes greater than 24 hours.
   C. chorioamnionitis.
   D. sibling with previous neonatal GBS infection.
   E. maternal GBS urinary tract infection.

6. **The following conditions have autosomal dominant inheritance:**
   A. achondroplasia.
   B. Huntington's chorea.
   C. Christmas disease.
   D. myotonia dystrophica.
   E. tuberous sclerosis.

7. **The following are side-effects of sulphasalazine:**
   A. reversible neutropenia.
   B. acute pancreatitis.
   C. methaemoglobinaemia.
   D. permanent oligospermia.
   E. folate deficiency.

8. **Insulin has the following effects:**
   A. decreased intracellular potassium.
   B. increased glycogen synthesis.
   C. increased fatty acid synthesis.
   D. decreased ketogenesis.
   E. decreased cell growth.

5. **ABCDE**
    Risk factors for neonatal GBS sepsis are:

    preterm labour
    rupture of membranes >18 hours prior to birth
    maternal chorioamnionitis
    maternal colonization with GBS
    previous baby with GBS sepsis
    maternal GBS urinary tract infection.

6. **ABDE**
    Autosomal dominant diseases include:

    achondroplasia
    adult polycystic kidney disease
    Gilbert's disease
    Hereditary spherocytosis
    Huntington's chorea
    hyperlipidaemia (type IV)
    Marfan's syndrome
    myotonic dystrophy
    neurofibromatosis
    retinoblastoma
    tuberous sclerosis
    von Willebrand's disease.

7. **ABCE**
    Sulphasalazine is a chemical combination of sulphapyridine
    and 5-aminosalicylic acid (5-ASA) and is useful in the treatment
    of ulcerative colitis. 5-ASA is the active moiety and sulphapyr-
    idine acts as a carrier to the colonic site of action. Common
    side-effects are nausea, vomiting, epigastric pain, headache and
    rash, occasionally fever, anaemia, reversible neutropenia, folate
    deficiency and reversible oligospermia. Rarer side-effects
    include methaemoglobinaemia, pancreatitis, hepatitis, throm-
    bocytopenia, agranulocytosis, aplastic anaemia and Stevens–
    Johnson syndrome.

8. **BCD**
    Insulin rapidly increases transport of glucose, amino acids and
    potassium into cells. It promotes glycogen synthesis, protein
    synthesis and lipogenesis. Hepatic ketogenesis is decreased.
    Insulin acts as a growth factor to all insulin-sensitive cells.

9. **A neonate is born with a supraventricular tachycardia which had been diagnosed antenatally. It has a blood pressure of 30/10, an enlarged liver and a pulse rate of 220/min. The following statements regarding management of the baby are correct:**
   A. vagatonic manoeuvres are not appropriate in this situation.
   B. adenosine is the intravenous treatment of choice.
   C. DC cardioversion at 10 J/kg may be used.
   D. intravenous verapamil and propranolol may be of use in this situation.
   E. in one-third of cases of SVT there is an underlying congenital cardiac lesion.

10. **In statistics:**
    A. increasing sample size widens the confidence intervals.
    B. the standard error (SE) is a measure of precision.
    C. the equation for a population regression line is $y = A + Bx$ where y is the independent variable.
    D. a Kaplan–Meier curve is the recognized way of showing survival curves.
    E. Mann-Whitney U-test is a parametric statistical test.

11. **Erythema nodosum:**
    A. is characterized by red, tender nodules over the forearm.
    B. is a recognized feature of tuberculosis.
    C. commonly occurs in inflammatory bowel disease.
    D. may be associated with viral infections.
    E. is characterized by target lesions.

12. **The following statements relating to the development of the human brain are correct:**
    A. the primitive brain vesicle appears at the end of the 4th week.
    B. the cerebral hemispheres result from evagination of the prosencephalon.
    C. the diencephalon is adjacent to the IIIrd ventricle.
    D. the cerebellum starts as a projection into the IVth ventricle.
    E. the nervous system develops from the ventral ectoderm at about the 16th day.

9. **BE**

   Although in this situation it is unlikely that vagal stimulation would stop the arrhythmia, it is worth attempting unilateral carotid massage even when there is evidence that the infant is in a haemodynamically compromised state. Adenosine at a starting dose of 50 μg/kg can be very effective at rapidly converting an SVT rhythm to a normal sinus rhythm. It works by slowing conduction through the A-V node which interrupts re-entry circuits. DC cardioversion at 0.5–1 J/kg can be extremely effective in returning the heart to a sinus rhythm, especially when the infant is in cardiac failure. Verapamil and propranolol should never be used together as hypotension and asystole can be precipitated. Verapamil is not recommended in children.

10. **D**

    As a sample size increases, the confidence intervals decrease in width. SE is a measure of imprecision. The equation for a population regression line is $y = A + Bx$ where y is the dependent variable and x the independent. The Mann-Whitney U-test is a non-parametric test. Its parametric equivalent is the Student's unpaired t-test.

11. **ABD**

    Erythema nodosum is characterized by red tender nodules over the tibia but may also appear on the thighs and forearms. Erythema nodosum is shiny and hot and can be surrounded by bruising. Causes include idiopathic, viral infections, streptococcal infections, ulcerative colitis and Crohn's disease. Erythema nodosum rarely occurs in inflammatory bowel disease. Target lesions refer to the rash seen with erythema multiforme.

12. **ABCD**

    Development of the brain begins with the appearance of the brain vesicles in the early part of the embryonic period. Evagination of the prosencephalon gives rise to the cerebral hemispheres. The primitive hemispheres and lamina terminalis constitute the telencephalon (endbrain). The diencephalon (epithalamus, thalamus and hypothalamic apparatus) is adjacent to the IIIrd ventricle. The cerebellum develops from a projection into the IVth ventricle. The nervous system develops from dorsal ectoderm at the 16th day. The neural tube begins to fuse at the end of the 3rd week. Rostral closure occurs on the 24th and caudal closure on the 26th day.

13. **The following are recognized causes of hypokalaemia:**
    A. Addison's disease.
    B. laxative abuse.
    C. liquorice ingestion.
    D. steroid therapy.
    E. metabolic acidosis.

14. **A diagnosis of immunodeficiency may be suggested by:**
    A. delayed separation of the umbilical cord.
    B. cerebellar ataxia.
    C. abscess formation in the neonatal period.
    D. albinism.
    E. failure to thrive, diarrhoea and respiratory infections.

15. **The following drugs are contraindicated in breast-feeding mothers:**
    A. bromocriptine.
    B. propranolol.
    C. digoxin.
    D. warfarin.
    E. tetracycline.

13. **BCD**

Causes of hypokalaemia are:

Increased urinary losses — loop diuretics
— steroids (iatrogenic, Cushing's syndrome)
— adrenocorticotrophic hormone (ACTH)
— renal failure (recovery from acute tubular necrosis)
— renal tubular acidosis
— liquorice (aldosterone-like effect)

Increased gut losses — vomiting
— diarrhoea
— laxative abuse

Redistribution — insulin/dextrose (for hyperkalaemia)
— alkalosis.

14. **ABCDE**

Delayed separation of the cord (with or without omphalitis) and abnormal scarring with serious infections are associated with LFA-1 deficiency. Cerebellar ataxia occurs in ataxia telangiectasia. The combination of partial albinism, an increased red reflex and recurrent bacterial infection suggests Chediak-Higachi syndrome. Combined immunodeficiency is characterized by diarrhoea, failure to thrive, pulmonary infections and cutaneous candidiasis.

15. **AE**

Bromocriptine suppresses lactation and should not be taken by breast-feeding mothers. Propranolol and digoxin are secreted in too small amounts to be harmful. There is a theoretical risk of haemorrhage in an infant if the mother is taking warfarin. This may especially be the case if the infant is deficient in vitamin K. However, in practice it is safe to use. Tetracycline will discolour the teeth of an infant and should be avoided.

16. **Hirschsprung's disease:**
    A. is confined to the rectum and sigmoid colon.
    B. often presents with large, hard stools.
    C. is a cause of acute enterocolitis in the neonatal period.
    D. is a recognized cause of diarrhoea in the neonatal period.
    E. is a recognized cause of failure to thrive.

17. **A normal baby of 12 months, born at term-would be expected to be able to:**
    A. get into a sitting position.
    B. build a tower of four bricks.
    C. have hearing reliably assessed using a distraction hearing test.
    D. feed with a spoon.
    E. point to eyes, nose and mouth.

18. **In bulimia nervosa:**
    A. male cases do not occur.
    B. weight is usually normal.
    C. dental problems are a recognized association.
    D. diabetes mellitus is a recognized association.
    E. the presence of amenorrhoea indicates a worse prognosis.

19. **Congenital heart disease may be associated with:**
    A. maternal diabetes.
    B. maternal smoking.
    C. maternal systemic lupus erythematosus (SLE).
    D. autosomal trisomies.
    E. intrauterine growth retardation (IUGR).

16. **CDE**

In most cases of Hirschsprung's disease the aganglionic segment is confined to the rectum and sigmoid colon, but in approximately 15% of cases may extend beyond the splenic flexure. Presentation in the neonatal period may be with delayed passage of first stool, incomplete intestinal obstruction (abdominal distension and vomiting, relieved by rectal stimulation and explosive release of watery stool) or with acute enterocolitis. Delayed presentation in childhood may occur. These children may have constipation, abdominal distension and failure to thrive.

17. **AC**

It is essential to have some knowledge of each of the four areas of child development (i.e. gross motor, fine motor and vision, hearing and speech and social behaviour) for several age groups. We suggest learning two to three normal milestones for each area of development for the following ages: 6 weeks, 6–8 months, 12 months, 18 months, 2½ years, 3 years, 4 years and 5 years.

18. **BCDE**

Bulimia nervosa is an eating disorder in which an intense preoccupation with food and weight is accompanied by episodes of binge eating and self induced vomiting. Over 90% of cases are female. Recurrent vomiting may cause erosion of dental enamel and a worse prognosis occurs in patients with menstrual irregularities, biochemical disturbances and concurrent depressive illness.

19. **ACD**

Maternal diabetes has many well-described effects on the fetus including an association with congenital heart disease. Maternal smoking is associated with an increase in the incidence of miscarriages, preterm labour, sudden infant death syndrome and small for gestational age infants. No effect on congenital heart disease has been clearly demonstrated. SLE is classically associated with congenital heart block. Mothers are usually positive to the anti-Rho antibody. The trisomies are commonly associated with congenital heart disease but there is no association with IUGR.

20. **During the first year of life in normal children, the percentage of body weight produced by the following decreases steadily:**
    A. total body water.
    B. intracellular fluid.
    C. extracellular fluid.
    D. fat.
    E. protein.

21. **The following signs can be present in a child with Asperger's syndrome:**
    A. significant language delay.
    B. stereotypical patterns of behaviour.
    C. lack of eye-to-eye contact.
    D. lack of ability to develop peer relationships.
    E. over 3 years old when symptoms start to develop.

22. **Abnormal sweat tests with chloride levels of >60 mmol/l can be seen in the following conditions:**
    A. ectodermal dysplasia.
    B. diabetes mellitus.
    C. nephrogenic diabetes insipidus.
    D. hypothyroidism.
    E. adrenal hypoplasia.

23. **Low levels of C3 can be seen in the following conditions:**
    A. chronic membranoproliferative glomerulonephritis.
    B. systemic lupus erythematosus (SLE).
    C. liver cirrhosis.
    D. dermatitis herpetiformis.
    E. hereditary angioedema.

20. ACD

The proportion of body weight provided by water may be more than 80% in preterm infants but falls to 72% by term. This gradually decreases to approximately 60% in adults. Although the proportion of body weight produced by fat increases in early infancy, there is a small net loss during the first year, while the percentage of protein increases slightly.

21. BCD

In childhood autism there are impairments in social interaction and communication. Repetitive activities are also present. In Asperger's syndrome there is normal cognitive and language development. However, in common with childhood autism there are sterotypical patterns of behaviour and marked social impairment. In both conditions the symptoms must have started before the age of 3 years.

22. ACDE

The sweat test is commonly used to diagnose cystic fibrosis. In the test pilocarpine is carried into the skin to induce sweating. At least 100 mg of sweat is needed for accurate measurements to be made. Conditions such as ectodermal dysplasia, nephrogenic diabetes insipidus, hypothyroidism and adrenal hypoplasia have increased electrolyte concentrations in sweat and may give false-positive results.

23. ABCD

In chronic membranoproliferative glomerulonephritis, SLE and dermatitis herpetiformis, the reduced levels of C3 are due to consumption of the factors by circulating immune complexes. The low level of C3 that is seen in severe liver cirrhosis is due to reduced synthesis. In hereditary angioedema low levels of C4 are present and the C3 levels are normal.

24. **The following statements are correct:**
    A. it is recommended that folate supplements should be taken by all pregnant women in order to prevent neural tube defects.
    B. the dose of folate necessary to prevent neural tube defects in a first pregnancy is 5 mg.
    C. pregnant women who are taking phenytoin may need to increase their dose of folate.
    D. the recommended dose of folate in a pregnant woman who has had a previous baby with a neural tube defect is 5 mg.
    E. supplementation with folate should continue throughout pregnancy.

25. **The following statements regarding lymphomas in childhood are correct:**
    A. Hodgkin's disease is more common than non-Hodgkin's under the age of 5 years.
    B. Hodgkin's disease has equal sex incidence.
    C. lymphocyte-predominant Hodgkin's disease has the worse prognosis.
    D. the nodular sclerosing variety is the most common form of Hodgkin's disease.
    E. the most common presenting clinical sign is splenomegaly.

26. **Immunoglobulin G (IgG):**
    A. crosses the placenta.
    B. is secreted in breast milk in significant quantities.
    C. levels decrease in preterm neonates after exchange transfusion.
    D. levels are lowest 4–6 months post-term.
    E. provides immunity to tuberculosis.

24. ACD

It has been proven that supplementing the diet with folate can prevent neural tube defects. Prevention in women in their first pregnancy should start in the preconception period. A dose of 400 µg is recommended and should be continued until the 12th week of pregnancy. In a woman who has previously had a baby with a neural tube defect a higher dose of 5 mg is recommended. Folate levels can be reduced in women on phenytoin. For this reason pregnant women on this medication should have an increased dose of folate.

25. D

Hodgkin's lymphoma occurs in four forms: (1) lymphocyte-predominant (10–20%) with the best prognosis; (2) nodular sclerosing (50%) which is the most common form; (3) mixed cellularity (40–50%) which is most likely to have extranodular disease at presentation; and (4) lymphocyte depleted (<10%) which is the rarest type with the worst prognosis. Hodgkin's disease is rarely found in children aged less than 5 years old (male:female ratio= 2:1) and peaks at between 15 and 34 years. Non-Hodgkin's disease is more common in younger children (male:female ratio= 3:1). The most common presenting clinical sign is enlarged cervical lymph nodes.

26. AD

Immunoglobulin G (IgG) crosses the placenta from as early as 12 weeks gestation. This is initially a slow process and transfer increases rapidly only after about 30 weeks gestation. Postnatal levels of IgG decline, reaching a nadir at approximately 4–6 months, until endogenous production becomes significant. The antibody content of colostrum and breast milk is almost entirely immunoglobulin A. Cell-mediated mechanisms provide immunity to tuberculosis.

27. **The following conditions characteristically present with hypoglycaemia and an absence of ketones in the urine:**
    A. multiple acyl CoA hydrogenase (MCAD) deficiency.
    B. proprionic acidaemia.
    C. urea cycle defects.
    D. tyrosinaemia.
    E. nesidioblastosis.

28. **A term infant has stridor and signs of respiratory distress at birth. The following are diagnostic possibilities:**
    A. laryngotracheobronchitis.
    B. choanal atresia.
    C. laryngeal web.
    D. acute epiglottitis.
    E. vascular ring.

29. **The following statements regarding aortic stenosis (AS) are correct:**
    A. AS occurs more commonly than pulmonary stenosis (PS).
    B. AS has an equal sex distribution.
    C. valvular AS is commonly due to a bicuspid valve.
    D. AS has a recognized association with sudden death.
    E. exercise restriction may be indicated.

27. AE

In normal infants undergoing fasting, fatty acids are liberated from adipose tissue. These enter the cytoplasm and are converted to acyl CoA esters. These are then transported across the mitochondrial membrane as carnitine esters, which are then transformed into CO_2 and ketones. These ketones are used by the brain in response to hypoglycaemia. In MCAD there is hypoglycaemia and a paradoxical lack of ketosis as the acyl CoA esters are not produced. In proprionic acidaemia there is a acidosis and hypoglycaemia accompanied by ketonuria. In nesidioblastosis there is hyperinsulinism resulting from a diffuse proliferation of the islet cells in the pancreas. Owing to the hyperinsulism there is hypoglycaemia with no ketogenesis.

28. BCE

Causes of upper airways obstruction in the newborn include:

  choanal atresia
  Pierre-Robin anomaly
  tracheal agenesis
  tracheal stenosis
  laryngomalacia
  laryngeal web
  vascular ring
  subglottic stenosis
  external compression (e.g. cystic hygroma).

29. CDE

AS is three times more common in males than females. Obstruction may be at the valvular, subvalvular or supravalvular level. Valvular AS is most commonly due to a bicuspid valve. Left ventricular hypertrophy can develop in more severe cases and chest pain and syncope may occur. Most cases are asymptomatic. If the stenosis is critical in the newborn infant, congestive heart failure develops. Sudden death occurs in 1–2% of children with severe AS. Exercise restriction is indicated in children with severe AS.

30. **The following statements regarding classical phenylketonuria (PKU) are correct:**
    A. eczema is characteristically present in young children with the disease.
    B. phenylalanine is not detectable in cord blood in newborn infants with PKU.
    C. dietary restrictions are stopped after the age of 10 years.
    D. a pregnant woman with PKU will not put her baby at risk if she is on an unrestricted diet.
    E. vomiting is an early presenting symptom of the disease.

31. **The following are recognized causes of neonatal cholestasis:**
    A. hepatitis B.
    B. cystic fibrosis.
    C. HIV infection.
    D. hypothyroidism.
    E. total parenteral nutrition (TPN).

30. ABE

Classical PKU is the result of a deficiency of phenylalanine hydroxylase. Eczema is often present in younger children, which disappears as the child grows older. Phenylalanine levels may rise to levels that are detectable by the Guthrie test as soon as 4 hours after birth, even before the ingestion of protein containing milk. It is recommended that a diet low in phenylalanine is continued for life. It has been shown that changes in white matter on stopping dietary restrictions are reversible on resumption of a low phenylalanine diet. It is essential that women with PKU should be on a diet low in phenylalanine in the preconception period to avoid damaging a normal fetus.

31. ABCDE

Conjugated hyperbilirubinaemia may result from cholestasis or increased bilirubin load. Causes of conjugated hyperbilirubinaemia in the newborn include:

intrauterine infections (Toxoplasmosis, Rubella, Cytomegalovirus and Herpes Simplex (TORCH), hepatitis B, syphilis, HIV)
sepsis
biliary atresia
paucity of intrahepatic bile ducts (Alagille's syndrome)
giant cell hepatitis
alpha-1-antitrypsin deficiency
bile plugs
long-term parenteral nutrition
choledochal cyst
cystic fibrosis
inborn errors of metabolism (galactosaemia, tyrosinosis, hypermethioninaemia)
hypothyroidism
Rotor syndrome
Dubin-Johnson syndrome
rhesus isoimmunization (post-exchange transfusion).

32. **The following statements about Hunter syndrome are correct:**
    A. corneal clouding is commonly found.
    B. inheritance is autosomal recessive.
    C. a child born with this condition appears normal at birth.
    D. hepatosplenomegaly is always present.
    E. diagnosis is confirmed by the presence of dermatan and heparan sulphate in the urine.

33. **The following statements regarding Lyme disease are correct:**
    A. erythema migrans is a pathognomonic feature of the disease.
    B. the infection is spread by sand flies.
    C. the infecting agent is a protozoa.
    D. a destructive arthritis can occur following infection.
    E. there is an increased risk of chronic disease-related symptoms in patients who are HLA-DR2.

34. **Noonan's syndrome has the following features:**
    A. neck webbing.
    B. low-set ears.
    C. chromosome 45XO.
    D. congenital subvalvular pulmonary stenosis.
    E. normal IQ in most cases.

35. **The following may occur after long-term, high-dose systemic steroid therapy:**
    A. hyponatraemia.
    B. osteoporosis.
    C. increased protein catabolism.
    D. increased appetite.
    E. neutropenia.

32. CD

Hunter syndrome is the only X-linked mucopolysaccharidosis disorder. Unlike Hurler syndrome, corneal clouding is rarely found. There is a severe manifestation of the syndrome, type A, and a milder form, type B. Children with both types are normal at birth. In type A, mental retardation is severe, hearing loss is common, and hepatosplenomegaly is present. The definitive diagnosis is made from iduronosulphate deficiency in the serum, cultured fibroblasts or white blood cells. Dermatan and heparan sulphate in the urine is common to both Hunter and Hurler syndrome.

33. ADE

Lyme disease is a tick-borne illness. Erythema migrans initially starts as a tick bite. This then develops into an annular erythematous lesion with central clearing. Similar secondary lesions then develop. The causative agent is the spirochaete *Borrelia burgdorferi*. Late manifestations of the disease can affect the central nervous system, cardiovascular system and/or musculoskeletal system.

34. AB

Noonan's syndrome occurs in both males and females. The karyotype is normal. Certain of the phenotypic features are the same as Turner's syndrome. Features of Noonan's syndrome include: short stature, neck webbing, pectus carinatum or excavatum, cubitus valgus, pulmonary valvular stenosis, atrial septal defect and a characteristic facies (hypertelorism, epicanthic folds, antimongolian slant to the eyes, ptosis, micrognathia and ear abnormalities). Cryptorchidism is common in the males and low IQ is more common than in Turner's syndrome.

35. BCD

High-dose systemic steroid therapy causes typical 'Cushingoid' features with moon face, thinning of hair, acne, thinning of skin, muscle wasting, redistribution of subcutaneous fat, striae and bruises. Catabolism of protein leads to an increase in amino acid conversion to glucose and contributes to hyperglycaemia. Salt and water retention occur and hypokalaemia may be present. Hypertension is common. Osteoporosis may lead to pathological fractures. Increased appetite, hyperactivity, insomnia or even psychosis may occur. Total white blood cell count and neutrophil count usually increase.

36. A 3-year-old child presents to hospital with a 10-day history of abdominal pain and bloody diarrhoea. On examination the child appears anaemic and jaundiced. The following laboratory findings are consistent with a diagnosis of haemolytic uraemic syndrome (HUS):
    A. positive Coombs' test.
    B. normal osmotic fragility test.
    C. low reticulocyte count and anaemia.
    D. increased fibrin degradation products.
    E. raised lactate dehydrogenase levels in the serum.

37. The following statements regarding an atrioventricular septal defect (AVSD) are correct:
    A. most defects occur in children with Down's syndrome.
    B. congestive heart failure usually occurs by 4–8 weeks of age.
    C. without surgical treatment most infants will die between the ages of 2 and 3 years.
    D. an ECG rarely shows right ventricular hypertrophy (RVH) or right bundle branch block (RBBB).
    E. a loud 3-4/6 pansystolic murmur is audible along the left sternal edge (LSE).

36. BDE

HUS is the most common cause of acute renal failure in an otherwise healthy child. It presents with a bloody diarrhoea that may have been present for 1–3 weeks. *E. coli* O157:H7 is the most commonly implicated organism. Anaemia results from haemolysis of red blood cells (RBC) in the microvasculature. Laboratory findings include: reticulocytosis, unconjugated hyperbilirubinaemia, increased lactate dehydrogenase (released from RBC), decreased haptoglobulins, a negative Coombs' test and normal red cell enzymes and osmotic fragility. A neutrophil leucocytosis usually occurs. If the leucocytosis is > 20×10^9/l, there is a poorer prognosis.

37. BCE

AVSDs account for about 2% of all congenital heart disease. Children with Down's syndrome only account for about 30% of all AVSDs. Heart failure occurs early and requires aggressive medical treatment. Recurrent chest infections are common. Surgical intervention is essential for long-term survival. An ECG shows left anterior hemiblock (superior QRS axis), a QRS axis between $-40°$ and $-150°$. RVH or RBBB is present in all patients and left ventricular hypertrophy may occur. First-degree atrioventricular block with a prolonged PR interval is also common.

38. **Causes of neonatal thrombocytopenia include:**
    A. intrauterine hypoxia.
    B. Henoch-Schonlein purpura.
    C. von Willebrand's disease.
    D. maternal systemic lupus erythematosus (SLE).
    E. necrotizing enterocolitis.

39. **The following statements are true:**
    A. Erb's palsy is due to damage to the radial nerve.
    B. the radial nerve supplies the skin on the radial side of the palm of the hand.
    C. the nerve roots of the radial nerve are C4–C6.
    D. the radial nerve supplies the 3rd and 4th lumbrical muscles.
    E. the radial nerve can be damaged by a fracture of the shaft of the humerus.

40. **Adenovirus is a recognized cause of the following childhood illnesses:**
    A. gastroenteritis.
    B. pneumonia.
    C. otitis media.
    D. obliterative bronchiolitis.
    E. high-grade fever without focus of infection.

38. ADE

Causes of neonatal thrombocytopenia:

maternal autoimmune thrombocytopenia
maternal isoimmune thrombocytopenia
drug-induced (infant or maternal)
maternal SLE
sepsis
disseminated intravascular coagulation
consumption (large thrombus/haemorrhage)
giant haemangioma (Kasabach-Merritt syndrome)
necrotizing enterocolitis
congenital viral infection
hypersplenism
Wiscott-Aldrich syndrome (small, abnormal platelets)
Bernard-Soulier syndrome (large, abnormal platelets)
marrow infiltration (malignancy, storage disease)
congenital abnormalities [Thrombocytopenia Absent Radius
    (TAR) syndrome, Fanconi's anaemia]
rhesus isoimmunization
post-exchange transfusion.

39. E

Erb's palsy occurs as a result of damage to the brachial plexus, injuring the C5 and C6 nerve roots, after downward traction on the arm. The radial nerve is the main branch of the posterior cord of the brachial plexus and has C5, 6, 7, 8 and T1 nerve roots. The skin supplied by the radial nerve is the lateral side of the dorsum of the hand.

40. ABCDE

Adenovirus may cause the following childhood illnesses:

upper respiratory tract infection
keratoconjunctivitis
otitis media
acute bronchiolitis
obliterative bronchiolitis
pneumonia
diarrhoea
meningitis
encephalitis
hepatitis
urinary tract infection
non-specific febrile illness.

41. **The following findings in the first week of life require investigation:**
    A. erythema toxicum neonatorum.
    B. subconjunctival haemorrhage.
    C. a bulging fontanelle.
    D. failure to pass meconium in the first 48 hours in a term infant.
    E. a squint.

42. **Hypersecretion of gastric acid is associated with:**
    A. duodenal ulcer.
    B. vagotomy.
    C. short bowel syndrome.
    D. Zollinger-Ellison syndrome.
    E. ranitidine.

43. **The following viral infections are paired with their appropriate incubation periods:**
    A. measles   –   10–12 days.
    B. rubella   –   7–14 days.
    C. Varicella zoster –   7–10 days.
    D. mumps   –   14–24 days.
    E. hepatitis B   –   60–110 days.

44. **Suicide in children:**
    A. is rare in children under 10 years old.
    B. is more common in girls than boys.
    C. is related to low self-esteem.
    D. is more commonly seen in children where there is a family history of affective disorders.
    E. is seen in children with poor impulse control.

41. CD

Erythema toxicum is a common rash of unknown aetiology which does not require investigation. Conjunctival haemorrhages commonly result from birth trauma and are frequently seen in the first week of life. A bulging fontanelle can be due to raised intracranial pressure, meningitis, intracranial bleeds or hydrocephalus. Most term infants pass meconium in the first 24 hours. Delay beyond this period can occur in cystic fibrosis, bowel atresia and Hirschsprung's disease. Full conjugate eye movement has usually developed by 6 months. In the first weeks of life squints are common and are usually of no consequence.

42. ACD

Gastric acid secretion is facilitated by parasympathetic stimulation via the vagus nerve in addition to local hormonal mechanisms mediated by gastrin. Duodenal ulceration is usually associated with hypersecretion of gastric acid whereas gastric ulceration often occurs with subnormal levels. Ranitidine inhibits gastric acid secretion by H_2 receptor antagonism. It is often useful in short bowel syndrome as hypergastrinaemia occurs in many cases leading to excessive gastric acid secretion. In Zollinger-Ellison syndrome there is hypersecretion of the gastrin-secreting cells of the antrum of the stomach. This leads to increased gastric acid secretion causing multiple peptic ulcers.

43. ADE

The incubation period of rubella is 14–21 days. Varicella zoster virus has an incubation period of 13–17 days.

44. ACDE

Suicide is rarely seen before the age of 10 years but the incidence is rising. The suicide rate is twice as high in boys compared with girls. The ratio is reversed in the incidence rate of attempted suicide. A family history of depression increases the risk of suicide. Over 50% of children who successfully commit suicide are said to have had impulsive personalities.

45. **A child presents with a left-sided ptosis, miosis and lack of sweating on the left side of his face. The following statements are correct:**
    A. these clinical signs are often associated with diminished tendon reflexes.
    B. investigations should include a chest X-ray.
    C. the site of the lesion must be distal to the superior cervical ganglion.
    D. if the pupil dilates with instillation of 4% cocaine solution, the site of the lesion is in the central nervous system.
    E. if the pupil dilates with instillation of 1:1000 adrenaline, the site of the lesion must be in the central nervous system.

46. **Features of coeliac disease include:**
    A. sensitivity to glutinin fraction of wheat protein.
    B. finger clubbing.
    C. disaccharidase deficiency.
    D. iron deficiency anaemia.
    E. crypt hypoplasia of small bowel mucosa.

47. **The following statements regarding dental development are correct:**
    A. calcification of the teeth starts in the seventh month of fetal life.
    B. in most children, deciduous teeth have started to erupt by 12 months.
    C. the first permanent teeth to erupt are molars.
    D. eruption of deciduous teeth can be delayed in hypothyroidism.
    E. calcification of permanent teeth starts at 2 years.

45. BD

The combination of these clinical signs indicate that the child has a Horner syndrome affecting the left side of his face. Horner syndrome is relatively common because of the long intra- and extracranial course of the sympathetic nerve fibres. As tumours or other compressive lesions may cause Horner syndrome, a chest X-ray is a mandatory part of the investigation of this problem. Diminished tendon reflexes are seen in association with the Holmes-Adie pupil. In this condition there is little or no pupillary reaction to light. Lesions distal to the superior cervical ganglion do not affect sweating. If the Horner syndrome is due to a lesion of the peripheral sympathetic tract, the pupil does not dilate in response to cocaine and dilates in response to adrenaline.

46. BCD

Coeliac disease is an immune-mediated hypersensitivity to the gliadin fraction of wheat and rye protein. Secondary disacchar-idase deficiency (usually lactase) may occur as a result of mucosal damage. Finger clubbing is a rare manifestation. Anaemia is more common in coeliac disease presenting in older children and may be due to iron or folate deficiency. Small intestinal biopsy shows mucosa with flat villi, crypt hyperplasia and lymphocytic infiltration of the lamina propria.

47. AD

Calcification of teeth begins in the 7th month of fetal life. Initially this is seen in the deciduous teeth until shortly before term when calcification of permanent teeth begins. In most infants eruption of deciduous teeth has started by 6 months although this can be delayed by factors such as malnutrition and hypothyroidism.

48. **The following statements are true:**
    A. the presence of hepatitis B surface antigen (HBsAg) indicates present infection or carrier status.
    B. babies born to mothers who are hepatitis B 'e' antibody (HBeAb) positive should be given hepatitis B immunoglobulin.
    C. hepatitis B vaccine and hepatitis B immunoglobulin are usually given in the same injection.
    D. babies born to mothers who are HBsAg positive and hepatitis B 'e' antigen (HBeAg) negative do not require hepatitis B vaccine.
    E. hepatitis B vaccine contains inactivated hepatitis B surface antigen.

49. **Poor prognostic factors in a child with acute lymphocytic leukaemia include:**
    A. B cell leukaemia.
    B. common ALL phenotype.
    C. a white cell count of $>50 \times 10^9$.
    D. age of diagnosis between 2 and 5 years.
    E. central nervous system disease at diagnosis.

50. **In X-linked recessive disorders the following statements are true:**
    A. only males are affected by the disorder.
    B. it is possible for the healthy son of a carrier to transmit the disorder.
    C. 50% of daughters of an affected male will be carriers.
    D. heterozygote females do not show signs of the disorder.
    E. none of the sons of an affected male will be affected.

51. **Maternal cocaine use in pregnancy has the following recognized effects:**
    A. increased incidence of preterm labour.
    B. uterine vessel vasoconstriction.
    C. placental abruption.
    D. marked neonatal withdrawal symptoms.
    E. fetal cardiac anomalies.

48. AE

The presence of HBsAg indicates present infection or carrier status. Mothers who are found to be HBsAg positive by antenatal testing should be screened for the presence of hepatitis B 'e' antigen (HBeAg) and hepatitis B 'e' antibody (HBeAb). Babies born to mothers found to be HBsAg positive should receive hepatitis B vaccine soon after birth and two further doses over the next 6–7 months. The presence of HBeAg without HBeAb confers a high risk of infection to the baby. These babies should receive hepatitis B vaccine as above, along with one dose of hepatitis B immunoglobulin, which is given within 48 hours of birth at a different site to the vaccination. Hepatitis B vaccine is made using recombinant DNA technology and contains inactivated HBsAg.

49. ACE

Poor prognostic factors in acute lymphocytic leukaemia also include an age of less than 1 year at diagnosis and the presence of a 4:11 translocation in malignant cells.

50. E

In X-linked recessive disorders only the males are affected although heterozygote females may show some signs of the condition. It is not possible for a healthy male to transmit the disorder. All the daughters of an affected male will be obligate carriers of the condition, but none of the sons.

51. ABC

Cocaine blocks noradrenaline reuptake at pre-synaptic receptors of alpha adrenergic neurons. This leads to uterine vessel vasoconstriction, resulting in decreased uterine blood flow, fetal hypoxia and increased fetal blood pressure. Fetal vasospasm may occur resulting in digit loss or cerebral infarction. The fetal hypoxia contributes to intrauterine growth retardation. An increased incidence of early pregnancy loss occurs, along with placental abruption and preterm labour. Unlike opiates, cocaine is not usually associated with a marked neonatal withdrawal reaction.

52. **Antidiuretic hormone (ADH):**
    A. is stored in the anterior pituitary gland.
    B. release is stimulated by hypernatraemia.
    C. release is inhibited by hypotension.
    D. release is stimulated by mannitol.
    E. leads to water reabsorption by increasing the water permeability of the ascending loop of Henle.

53. **In children with cystic fibrosis:**
    A. serum immunoreactive trypsin is decreased in the first 2 weeks of life.
    B. the concentration of sweat chloride is usually greater than that of sodium.
    C. pneumonia is the most common presentation in the neonatal period.
    D. a large appetite is a common feature in infancy.
    E. Bartter's syndrome is a recognized feature.

54. **The following are correct associations:**
    A. basophilic stippling   – folate deficiency.
    B. Diamond-Blackfan syndrome – hypercellular marrow.
    C. aplastic anaemia   – phenytoin.
    D. lymphopenia   – Wiskott-Aldrich syndrome.
    E. decreased megakaryocytes   – Idiopathic thrombocyto-penia purpura (ITP).

52. **BD**

ADH is a peptide hormone that is synthesized in the hypothalamus and stored in the posterior pituitary. Release is mainly stimulated by increased plasma osmolality, which may be secondary to hypernatraemia, hyperglycaemia or mannitol therapy. When plasma volume decreases significantly, non-osmotic stimulation of ADH secretion occurs via aortic and left atrial baroreceptors. ADH increases the water permeability of the renal medullary collecting ducts, thus leading to the formation of concentrated urine. The ascending loop of Henle is impermeable to water.

53. **BD**

An elevated immunoreactive trypsin (IRT) is found in neonates with cystic fibrosis and this may be used as a diagnostic test. In children with cystic fibrosis the sweat chloride is greater than the sweat sodium and the sum of these exceeds 140 mmol/l. The opposite applies for normal individuals. The most common presentation in the neonatal period is with meconium ileus, which occurs in approximately 10–15% of cases. Cystic fibrosis may present in infancy with failure to thrive but appetite is usually noted to be particularly good. Pseudo-Bartter's syndrome may occur as a result of excessive sweat sodium and potassium loss.

54. **CD**

Haematological finding	Cause/condition
Basophilic stippling	Defective erythropoiesis, lead poisoning
Hypoplastic anaemia	Diamond-Blackfan syndrome, autoimmune causes, penicillin, barbiturates, chloramphenicol, phenytoin, mumps, mycoplasma, parvovirus, leukaemia, chronic renal failure
Aplastic anaemia	Fanconi's anaemia, idiopathic, radiation, cytotoxics, carbamazepine, carbimazole, chloramphenicol, chlorpromazine, ethosuximide, penicillin
Lymphopenia ($<2.0 \times 10^9$/l)	Aplastic anaemia, Wiskott-Aldrich syndrome, SCIDS, HIV
Thrombocytopenia ($<150\,000$/mm^3)	ITP, Fanconi's anaemia, thrombocytopenia with absent radius, HUS, Wiskott-Aldrich syndrome, DIC, leukaemia, radiation, cytoxics, sodium valproate, hypersplenism, congenital CMV/rubella.

SCIDS, severe combined immunodeficiency syndrome; DIC, disseminated intravascular coagulation; CMV, cytomegalovirus; HUS, haemolytic uraemic syndrome.

55. **The following conditions show characteristic changes on an electroencephalogram (EEG):**
   A. Angleman syndrome.
   B. infantile spasms.
   C. subacute sclerosing panencephalitis (SSPE).
   D. petit mal seizures.
   E. multiple sclerosis.

56. **In human skin:**
   A. anagen is the active phase of hair growth.
   B. ultraviolet light is important in the conversion of 7-dehydrocholesterol (7-DHCC) to cholecalciferol (CC).
   C. nuclei and cell organelles are lost in the prickle cell layer.
   D. the paccinian corpuscles detect pressure.
   E. lanugo hair appears at 20 weeks gestation but usually largely disappears before birth.

57. **The neonatal electrocardiogram:**
   A. has an axis shifted to the right in preterm infants.
   B. sinus arrhythmia is normal in term infants.
   C. R-wave in lead V_1 > 20 mm indicates right ventricular hypertrophy (RVH).
   D. S-wave in lead V_1 > 20 mm indicates left ventricular hypertrophy (LVH).
   E. a short PR interval is associated with a supraventricular tachycardia.

58. *Helicobacter pylori:*
   A. is associated with antral gastritis.
   B. colonizes the mucosa primarily.
   C. is only a minor factor in gastric ulceration.
   D. may be treated with a combination of bismuth and antibiotics.
   E. is not of importance in the origin of intestinal ulcers in childhood.

55. ABCD

In Angleman syndrome a characteristic rhythmic delta wave pattern is present on the EEG. Infantile spasms show a hypsarrthymic pattern on the EEG with a multifocal high voltage spike and slow waves present in over 60% of infants with the condition. SSPE has regular repeated bursts of high voltage slow waves on the EEG. The EEG in petit mal epilepsy shows spike and wave discharges at the rate of 3 Hz.

56. ABDE

The three phases of hair growth are anagen (active), catagen (rest) and telogen (shedding). Following pregnancy a large number of hair cells shed: telogen effluvium. UV light is important for the conversion of 7-DHCC to CC in the skin. 1-hydroxylation (1-OH vitamin D) occurs in the kidney and 25-hydroxylation (1,25-OH vitamin D) occurs in the liver. Liver and/or kidney disease can impair vitamin D metabolism. Loss of nuclei and cell organelles occurs in the granular layer. Paccinian corpuscles detect pressure and Meissner's corpuscles detect touch. The fine body hair, lanugo, has largely disappeared by birth. Hair that covers the body is called velus and that on the scalp, eyebrows, beard, axilla and pubic areas is called terminal.

57. BCDE

The axis is shifted to the right in term neonates (mean +110–135 degrees). The same does not hold true for the preterm infant. Sinus arrhythmia is commonly found in term neonates. An R-wave > 20 mm in V_1 indicates RVH. An S-wave in lead V_1 > 20 mm indicates LVH. A supraventricular tachycardia can be associated with a short PR interval.

58. AD

Helicobacter pylori primarily colonizes the mucous layer above the mucosa and plays an important role in peptic ulceration in both adults and children. Treatment of peptic ulceration should be accompanied by eradication of associated *H. pylori* infection. The ideal treatment is unclear. Options include: (1) amoxycillin + metronidazole + tripotassium dicitratobismuthate; (2) amoxycillin + metronidazole + ranitidine; (3) amoxycillin + omeprazole. If necessary clarithromycin can be substituted for amoxycillin.

59. **The proximal renal tubule:**
    A. absorbs up to 20% of the glomerular filtrate.
    B. reabsorbs sodium via a passive process involving the consumption of ATP.
    C. reabsorbs glucose via a co-transport process with sodium.
    D. actively secretes hydrogen ions into the urine.
    E. does not reabsorb water.

60. **The following are associated with neonatal hypoglycaemia:**
    A. Down's syndrome.
    B. Reye syndrome.
    C. nesidioblastosis.
    D. galactosaemia
    E. polycythaemia.

59. CD
The proximal renal tubule reabsorbs up to 65% of the glomerular filtrate. Sodium transport is driven by an active process driven by the consumption of ATP. Glucose and amino acids are reabsorbed in a co-transport system with sodium. Up to 65% of water is reabsorbed by the proximal renal tubule.

60. CDE
Causes of neonatal hypoglycaemia can be classified as follows:

Hyperinsulinism	– maternal diabetes
	– islet cell hyperplasia
	– Beckwith-Wiedemann syndrome
	– nesidioblastosis
	– islet cell adenoma
Decreased production	– prematurity
	– intrauterine growth retardation
	– glycogen storage disease
	– galactosaemia
Increased utilization	– hypothermia
	– polycythaemia
	– asphyxia
	– sepsis
Inborn errors	– maple syrup urine disease (MSUD)
	– proprionic acidaemia
	– methylmalonic acidaemia
	– tyrosinaemia
Endocrine causes	– panhypopituitarism
	– adrenal insufficiency
Miscellaneous	– maternal drugs (beta agonists/ blockers, thiazides)
	– post-exchange transfusion.

Paper 2

1. **Proximal (type II) renal tubular acidosis (RTA):**
   A. occurs in cystinosis.
   B. results in less bicarbonate loss than that seen in distal (type I) RTA.
   C. results in hypochloraemic alkalosis.
   D. hypokalaemia if present is mild.
   E. may result from an acquired Fanconi syndrome.

2. **The following statements are true:**
   A. peripheral blood contains approximately 500 times as many red cells as white cells.
   B. red blood cells have a shorter lifespan than neutrophils.
   C. differentiation of lymphocyte precursors into B-cells occurs mainly in the thymus.
   D. B-lymphocytes produce humoral immunity.
   E. bursal equivalents in humans include fetal liver and bone marrow.

3. **The following childhood infections are paired with an appropriate antibiotic treatment:**
   A. amoxycillin   – acute epiglottitis.
   B. erythromycin   – Lyme disease.
   C. tetracycline   – *Chlamydia* pneumonia.
   D. ceftriaxone   – Meningococcal meningitis.
   E. benzyl penicillin – neonatal *Listeria* septicaemia.

4. **The following statements regarding a retinoblastoma are correct:**
   A. patients can present with strabismus.
   B. tumours spontaneously regress in 10% of cases.
   C. all bilateral cases of retinoblastoma are hereditary.
   D. patients with a family history of retinoblastoma have a 25% chance of transmitting the disease to their children.
   E. other types of malignancies develop in 15% of children.

1. **AE**

   Proximal RTA results from reduced proximal tubular reabsorption of bicarbonate. Bicarbonate loss is greater than in distal RTA. Hypokalaemia results from sodium reabsorption and flooding the distal tubule with sodium bicarbonate. Extracellular fluid (ECF) volume contraction occurs as a result of sodium loss, which stimulates chloride reabsorption causing a hyperchloraemia. Decreased ECF worsens hypokalaemia because of increased aldosterone secretion. Heavy metal poisoning (lead, magnesium, cadmium) can produce a Fanconi syndrome.

2. **ADE**

   The lifespan of neutrophils is very short (only several hours), whereas red blood cells survive for an average of 120 days. T-lymphocytes differentiate in the thymus and B-lymphocytes differentiate in bursal equivalent tissue, which in humans includes bone marrow and fetal liver.

3. **D**

   Acute epiglottitis is most commonly caused by *Haemophilus influenza* which may be resistant to amoxycillin. It is therefore best treated with either chloramphenicol or a third-generation cephalosporin. Lyme disease is caused by the spirochaete *Borrellia burgdorferi* which is sensitive to penicillin. Chlamydial infections should be treated with erythromycin in children. Tetracycline is contraindicated in children because it discolours the teeth. Meningococcal meningitis may be treated with a one-daily dose of ceftriaxone. The treatment of choice for *Listeria* infections in neonates is ampicillin.

4. **ACE**

   The most common presentation of a retinoblastoma is with a white reflex. Tumours regress in about 1% of cases and for this reason the parents of a child with the disease should have their eyes examined for signs of retinal scarring. This is important as the tumour is inherited in up to 15% of unilateral tumours. The gene mutation that results in the tumour developing is on chromosome 13q. The inheritance is autosomal dominant with incomplete penetrance and around 80% of children with the abnormal gene develop a retinoblastoma. The most common malignancy is osteogenic sarcoma of the femur.

5. **The following are recognized causes of conjugated hyperbilirubinaemia in the newborn:**
   A. alpha thalassaemia.
   B. maternal blood group A Rhesus positive, baby's blood group O Rhesus positive.
   C. galactosaemia.
   D. Gilbert's syndrome.
   E. cystic fibrosis.

6. **The following statements regarding Rett syndrome are true:**
   A. it is only seen in girls.
   B. mental handicap is rarely present.
   C. fits are common.
   D. macrocephaly is always present.
   E. respiratory failure is often the cause of death.

7. **Deficiency of cell mediated immunity occurs in the following:**
   A. agammaglobulinaemia.
   B. asthma.
   C. human immunodeficiency virus (HIV) infection.
   D. malnutrition.
   E. Di George syndrome.

8. **A 2-year-old child with tetralogy of Fallot presents in the process of having a cyanotic spell. The following statements are correct:**
   A. cyanotic attacks are more common at night.
   B. intravenous propranolol may terminate an attack.
   C. digoxin may help prevent further spells happening.
   D. the systolic murmur characteristically increases during a spell.
   E. squatting during a spell increases systemic vascular resistance and increases blood supply to the lungs.

9. **A baby born at 42 weeks gestation has a birth weight of 4.3 kg. At 1 hour of age the serum glucose is found to be 0.5 mmol. The following are possible causes for the hypoglycaemia:**
   A. post-maturity.
   B. maternal hypertension.
   C. maternal gestational diabetes.
   D. Beckwith-Wiedemann syndrome.
   E. nesidioblastosis.

5. **CE**

   See Question 31, Paper 1.

6. **ACE**

   Rett syndrome is only seen in girls as it is fatal in male fetuses. Postnatal microcephaly is present and development reaches a plateau and then regresses. Severe mental handicap is always present. Typical features also include hand wringing, teeth grinding and panting. Seizures are often present and, as the disease progresses, spasticity develops. Respiratory failure resulting from scoliosis is a common cause of death in children affected by this disorder.

7. **CDE**

   Causes of deficient cell mediated immunity include:

   severe combined immune deficiency (SCID)
   defects of neutrophil mobility/chemotaxis
   Di George syndrome
   malnutrition
   post-infection (e.g. measles)
   cancer chemotherapy
   HIV infection.

8. **BE**

   The systolic murmur in tetralogy of Fallot is due to the obstruction of right ventricular outflow, usually as a result of infundibular narrowing. Cyanotic spells occur as a result of infundibular spasm. The murmur decreases in intensity, there is an alteration in the level of consciousness and a sudden onset of dyspnoea. Cyanotic spells tend to occur in the morning. Squatting increases systemic vascular resistance and decreases the return of deoxygenated venous blood from the legs. This helps reduce the oxygen debt that occurs during a spell. Digoxin therapy is contraindicated because it increases infundibular spasm. Spells can be treated with oxygen, placing the patient in the knee–chest position, giving morphine 0.1 mg/kg and propranolol at 0.1 mg/kg.

9. **CDE**

   See Question 60, Paper 1.

10. **A 5-year-old child presents with progressive weakness. The following make a diagnosis of Guillain-Barré syndrome more likely:**
    A. isolation of *Campylobacter jejuni* from the stool.
    B. leg pain.
    C. dilated pupils.
    D. the presence of over 50 lymphocytes/ml in the cerebrospinal fluid (CSF).
    E. asymmetric weakness of the lower limbs.

11. **Causes of grossly elevated erythrocyte sedimentation rate (ESR) (> 100 mm/hour) include:**
    A. polycythaemia rubra vera (PRV).
    B. hypofibrinoginaemia.
    C. systemic lupus erythematosus.
    D. uraemia.
    E. profound anaemia.

12. **The following statements are true:**
    A. confidence intervals can only be applied to normal data.
    B. large confidence intervals show that a study is of no clinical use.
    C. the Wilcoxon paired test is used in non-parametric analysis.
    D. standard deviations can only be calculated for normal populations.
    E. the standard error of the mean is always less than the standard deviation.

13. **Concerning the development of the cardiovascular system:**
    A. the main pulmonary artery develops from the left 6th branchial arch.
    B. a right-sided aortic arch is usually present at 10 weeks.
    C. the ductus arteriosus is the dorsal remnant of the right-sided aortic arch.
    D. the septum secundum grows up as a limbus of the foramen ovale.
    E. atrioventricular septal defects (AVSD) may involve defects of the septum primum.

10. **AB**

Guillain-Barré syndrome (GBS) has been shown to be associated with *C. jejuni* infection. Pain is often a predominant feature of GBS and is the presenting symptom in up to 20% of cases. Children who present with pain often have significant emotional lability associated with vomiting and a headache. Pupillary abnormalities are not seen in GBS and when present suggest diptheria or botulism. The presence of over 50 lymphocytes/ml of CSF suggests polio or central nervous system lymphoma. In GBS the protein level in the CSF is typically 80–200 mg/dl. Paralysis of the lower limbs is usually symmetrical and is frequently associated with distal paresthesias and numbness.

11. **CDE**

There are many causes of an abnormal ESR.

(1) Increased ESR: dysproteinaemia, giant cell arteritis, sepsis, carcinomatosis, uraemia, profound anaemia.

(2) Decreased ESR: PRV, cryoglobulinaemia, profound hypogammaglobulinaemia.

12. **CDE**

Methods exist for calculating confidence intervals for non-parametric data. Even if confidence intervals are large they may indicate that a useful clinical response is present in the data and that larger trials may be indicated. As the standard error of the mean is standard deviation/n, it will always be smaller than the standard deviation.

13. **ABCDE**

The blood and cardiovascular system are derived from mesoderm and first appear in the middle of the 3rd week. Bilateral ventral tubes fuse and by 21 days there is a single ventral heart tube that begins to beat by about the 23rd day. By 28 days the definitive chambers of the heart are apparent. In the 5th week, septal ridges grow together to septate the heart. The septum primum appears as a crescent-shaped downward growth of the postero-superior wall of the common atrium. Before the septum primum is complete, small openings appear in the upper portion; these merge to form the ostium secundum. On the right of the septum primum the thicker septum secundum grows down. It becomes complete except for a defect that becomes the oval foramen.

14. **The following statements about haemoglobin electrophoresis are correct:**
    A. by 3 months of age the normal adult haemoglobin pattern is present.
    B. haemoglobin A is not present in the fetus.
    C. haemoglobin F is raised in beta thalassaemia trait.
    D. haemoglobin A_2 is raised in sickle cell disease.
    E. haemoglobin A_2 is raised in sickle-thalassaemia disease.

15. **The following conditions can present with chronic constipation:**
    A. diabetes mellitus.
    B. hypercalcaemia.
    C. hypothyroidism.
    D. coeliac disease.
    E. abetalipoproteinaemia.

16. **A normal child of 18 months would be expected to be able to do the following:**
    A. climb stairs in an adult fashion.
    B. draw a circle.
    C. point to eyes, nose and mouth when instructed to do so.
    D. speak in short sentences.
    E. eat with a spoon and fork.

17. **In children with Down's syndrome:**
    A. the infant is usually hypertonic.
    B. asthma is more common.
    C. most mothers are over 35 years of age.
    D. karyotyping is always indicated.
    E. brachycephaly is characteristic.

18. **The following statements regarding anorexia nervosa are correct:**
    A. anorexia nervosa is 10 times more common in girls than boys.
    B. hypothermia can be present in children suffering from this condition.
    C. levels of luteinizing hormone (LH) and follicle-stimulating hormone (FSH) are typically decreased.
    D. decreased levels of serum alkaline phosphatase are typically present.
    E. anorexia nervosa is more commonly seen in children whose parents are of socio-economic class 5 compared with those whose parents are of socio-economic class 1.

14. **CE**

The normal adult haemoglobin pattern is seen by 6–12 months of age. HbA, in small amounts, is detectable even in the smallest embryos. HbF and HbA_2 are raised in beta thalassaemia trait. In sickle cell disease no HbA is detectable, HbF is raised but the HbA_2 level is normal. In sickle-thalassaemia disease HbA_2 and HbF are raised. In this condition painful crises may occur.

15. **ABC**

Both diabetes mellitus and hypercalcaemia can present with constipation. This is due to the dehydration that accompanies these conditions. In hypothyroidism there is decreased gut motility. Coeliac disease and abetalipoproteinaemia are characteristically associated with diarrhoea.

16. **C**

See Question 17, Paper 1.

17. **DE**

Infants with Down's syndrome (trisomy 21) are commonly hypotonic at birth. Brachycephaly a consistent clinical feature. Owing to cases of Down's syndrome where a translocation has occurred, karyotyping should always be carried out in order to assess the recurrence risk in parents and other family members.

18. **ABD**

Anorexia nervosa is more common in children whose parents have a high socio-economic status. A typical patient will have lost more than 20% of her average body weight. Symptoms resulting from hypometabolism include: amenorrhoea, hypothermia, bradycardia and hypotension. Pancytopenia, anaemia, leukopenia and thrombocytopenia are commonly found. Serum levels of cholesterol may be increased whilst lower levels of albumin and alkaline phosphatase can be seen. Increased levels of LH and FSH seem to be related to changes in hypothalamic function.

19. **The normal total fluid intake required is:**
    A. 200 ml/kg/24 hours in a day 1 28-week-gestation infant.
    B. 55 ml/kg/24 hours in a 1-year-old child.
    C. 55 ml/kg/24 hours in adults.
    D. 60 ml/kg/24 hours in a day 1 term infant.
    E. 100 ml/kg/24 hours in a 4-year-old child.

20. **Human breast milk:**
    A. has a sodium concentration of >20 mmol/l.
    B. is associated with prolonged neonatal jaundice, and if so breast feeding must be discontinued.
    C. in infact feeding decreases the likelihood of developing atopic disease in childhood.
    D. has a lower carbohydrate content than cow's milk.
    E. has a lower casein to lactalbumin ratio than cow's milk.

21. **The following statements regarding inhaled nitric oxide (NO) therapy are correct:**
    A. NO reduces intrapulmonary shunting.
    B. NO causes pulmonary and systemic vasodilatation.
    C. NO combines with oxygen to form nitrogen dioxide.
    D. pulmonary toxicity results from formation of nitric and nitrous acids.
    E. when used therapeutically it should be administered at concentrations of 250 parts per million (ppm).

19. CDE

Normal fluid requirements (in ml/kg/24hours):

Preterm (day 1)	60–80
Term (day 1)	60
<6 months	150
1 year	125
4 years	105
10 years	80
15 years–adult	55.

20. CE

It is important to know about the basic composition of milks and in particular the main differences between human breast milk and unmodified cow's milk. In addition it is useful to know the composition of a common formula milk and a special preterm formula. Unmodified cow's milk has a high sodium content (>20 mmol/l), whereas in breast and standard formula milks this is low ($\approx$6 mmol/l). Cows milk also has a high concentration of potassium, calcium and phosphate. The preterm formulae have a higher sodium content ($\approx$14 mmol/l) and more calories, reflecting the increased sodium losses of preterm infants and their greater calorific requirements. Breast, standard formula and preterm formula milks have a higher carbohydrate and lower protein content than unmodified cow's milk. Breast milk is associated with neonatal jaundice since it contains oestrogens (3-alpha, 20-beta-pregnanediol) and non-esterified long chain fatty acids which inhibit glucuronyl-1-transferase. There is increasing evidence that breast feeding decreases the likelihood of developing atopic disease, particularly if the mother avoids consuming dairy products or other likely allergens.

21. ACD

NO is a potent vasodilator and when used as an inhaled therapy improves intrapulmonary shunting by preferentially vasodilating well-ventilated areas of the lung. A big advantage NO has over other agents used as pulmonary vasodilators (e.g. prostacyclin, tolazoline) is its lack of systemic effects. The lowest possible concentration of NO that produces a therapeutic effect should be used. In most cases this is < 20 ppm but < 10 ppm is safer.

22. **In acute bronchiolitis:**
    A. ribavirin is the treatment of choice for hospitalized cases.
    B. lung volume is usually decreased.
    C. bronchodilators are usually effective.
    D. feeding difficulties are common.
    E. upper airway obstruction is a common feature.

23. **Increased gastric emptying that may alter the rate of drug absorption is found in the following conditions:**
    A. coeliac disease.
    B. raised intracranial pressure.
    C. migraine.
    D. duodenal ulcer.
    E. gastric ulcer.

24. **Umbilical hernia in early childhood is a recognized feature of the following:**
    A. Down's syndrome.
    B. prematurity.
    C. Hurler's syndrome.
    D. obesity.
    E. hypothyroidism.

25. **A 3-year-old girl presents with her first febrile convulsion. The following information should be given to her parents:**
    A. febrile convulsions occur in 5% of children.
    B. she has a 5% chance of developing idiopathic epilepsy.
    C. she has a 25% chance of having a further febrile convulsion.
    D. phenobarbitone will prevent any further seizures occurring.
    E. preschool booster vaccinations should not be given.

22. **D**

Acute bronchiolitis presents in infancy with signs of respiratory distress, hyperinflation, inspiratory crackles and often wheezing. Feeding difficulties are common and most hospitalized cases require nasogastric feeds or intravenous fluids. Bronchodilators are often ineffective and ribavirin treatment is reserved for cases where underlying cardiopulmonary disease or immunological deficiency presents an increased risk of mortality from bronchiolitis.

23. **AD**

Gastric emptying is an important determinant of rate and sometimes extent of drug absorption. Increased gastric emptying is associated with coeliac disease, duodenal ulcer and gastroenterostomy. Decreased gastric emptying occurs with raised intracranial pressure, migraine, pyloric stenosis, trauma, severe pain, gastric ulcer and intestinal obstruction.

24. **ABCE**

Umbilical hernia is most common in black infants and preterm infants. It is also found in infants with hypothyroidism, Hurler's syndrome and Down's syndrome.

25. **AC**

Febrile convulsions can be seen between the ages of 6 months and 5 years; 75% of children will have only one seizure. The most important factor in predicting whether or not a child will have further seizures is a strong family history of febrile seizures in close relatives. The convulsions are usually tonic-clonic in nature. Prospective follow-up studies suggest that idiopathic epilepsy develops in about 2% of infants, which is four times the incidence of the population at large. Phenobarbitone treatment reduces the incidence of further fits but will not prevent seizures occurring. It should not be given after only one seizure.

26. **The following statements regarding insulin-dependent diabetes mellitus are correct:**
    A. there is an increased incidence in children with the HLA-DR3 marker.
    B. early morning hyperglycaemia should be treated with an increase in insulin dosage.
    C. 10% of newly diagnosed diabetics have anti-islet cell antibodies.
    D. usual daily insulin requirements in a newly diagnosed diabetic are about 10 units/kg/day.
    E. hyperlipidaemia is commonly found in ketoacidosis.

27. **The following cause bullous lesions in children:**
    A. pemphigus.
    B. pemphigoid.
    C. dermatitis herpetiformis.
    D. dermatomyositis.
    E. systemic lupus erythematosus.

28. **A term neonate is found to have a heart murmur on routine examination. The following make it less likely to be an innocent murmur:**
    A. the mother has diabetes mellitus.
    B. the mother has corrected tetralogy of Fallot.
    C. an accessory digit is found in the mother and baby.
    D. a diastolic murmur is present.
    E. the ventricular axis on the ECG is +150°.

26. **AE**

When HLA-DR3 or HLA-DR4 markers are present there is a two to three times increased risk of developing diabetes when compared with the average incidence of the disease in the general population. If both are present there is a 10 times increased risk of developing diabetes. Early morning hyperglycaemia may be the result of the Somogyi effect. This occcurs when excessive insulin is administered in the evening. There is a rebound hyperglycaemia caused by increased cortisol, growth hormone and catecholamines. Hyperlipidaemia may be present in ketoacidosis as a result of the lipolytic effect of glycogen, cortisol, growth hormone and catecholamines. At the onset of diabetes, or during recovery from ketoacidosis, the daily insulin requirements are usually 0.5–1.0 units/kg/day.

27. **ABC**

Examples of bullous lesions in children are:

> herpes simplex virus infection
> epidermolysis bullosa
> dermatitis herpetiformis
> pemphigus
> pemphigoid.

28. **ABD**

Family history of congenital heart disease increases the risk in other family members. Maternal congenital heart disease increases the risk in her children to approximately 5%. This is similar to the increased risk of congenital heart disease in infants of insulin-dependent diabetic mothers. Although up to 30% of children with congenital heart disease have other abnormalities, the presence of an accessory digit is a common inherited defect (usually autosomal dominant and in black families) and is not usually associated with any other problems. Innocent heart murmurs are systolic only, usually short and may vary with the position of the baby. The normal neonatal ECG has a ventricular axis between 110° and 180°.

29. **Serum ferritin levels:**
    A. reliably reflect total body iron stores.
    B. indicate iron deficiency before anaemia occurs.
    C. accurately detect iron overload.
    D. are not as reliable as Total Iron Binding Capacity (TIBC) for detection of iron deficiency.
    E. are affected by diurnal variation.

30. **A newborn infant has ambiguous genitalia. The following statements are true:**
    A. assignment of gender is primarily dependent on karyotype.
    B. if gonads are palpable they are likely to be testes.
    C. the infant should be raised as a boy in all cases of male pseudohermaphroditism.
    D. if the karyotype is 46XX, 21-hydroxylase deficiency is the most likely diagnosis.
    E. gonads that are discordant for the assigned gender should be removed.

31. **The following statements regarding Wiskott-Aldrich syndrome are correct:**
    A. Wiskott-Aldrich syndrome can present with a cerebral haemorrhage.
    B. thrombocytopenia is typically present.
    C. serum IgA and IgE levels are characteristically decreased.
    D. eczema is often present.
    E. there is an absence of serum isohaemagluttinins.

29. **ABC**
    Serum ferritin is in equilibrium with body iron stores and low
    levels indicate iron deficiency early and before the onset of
    anaemia. High levels are a reliable indicator of iron overload.
    Unlike serum iron and TIBC saturation (which are poor
    indicators of body iron stores), ferritin levels are not affected by
    diurnal variation.

30. **BDE**
    In cases of ambiguous genitalia the determination of sex for
    rearing should be primarily determined by the feasibility of
    anatomic reconstruction and appropriate hormonal treatment
    rather than karyotype. The broad categories of diagnosis are
    female pseudohermaphroditism (most commonly secondary to
    21-hydroxylase deficiency), male pseudohermaphroditism or
    true hermaphroditism (rare). Male pseudohermaphrodites
    may have disorders of testosterone synthesis or partial end-
    organ resistance to testosterone (incomplete testicular femin-
    ization). The latter should never be raised as males as they
    never virilize. Gonads that are either discordant for the
    assigned gender or dysgenetic are surgically removed to reduce
    the risk of later malignancy.

31. **ABDE**
    Wiskott-Aldrich syndrome is an X-linked recessive disorder
    which is characterized by eczema, thrombocytopenia and an
    abnormal immune response to infections. The immunodefi-
    ciency results from hypermetabolism of immunoglobulins and
    an impairment of T-cell function. IgA and IgE levels are raised
    whilst serum isohaemaglutinins are typically absent.

32. **In the normal kidney:**
    A. over 50% of filtered sodium is passively reabsorbed from the proximal tubule.
    B. sodium is actively reabsorbed in the ascending loop of Henle.
    C. aldosterone increases sodium reabsorption from the medullary collecting ducts.
    D. dietary sodium loading leads to an increase in the glomerular filtration rate.
    E. the maximum urine concentrating capacity is decreased in preterm infants.

33. **A false negative Mantoux test may be present in the following conditions:**
    A. miliary tuberculosis.
    B. sarcoidosis.
    C. autoimmune thyroiditis.
    D. 2 mg/kg/day prednisolone therapy.
    E. previous Mantoux test.

34. **The following statements regarding systemic lupus erythematosis (SLE) are correct:**
    A. when disease is active the levels of complements C3 and C4 are raised.
    B. when evidence of a mild nephritis is present, a renal biopsy is unnecessary.
    C. there is a female preponderance of 8:1.
    D. first manifestation of the disease may be idiopathic thrombocytopenia purpura.
    E. there is neurological involvement in about 10% of cases.

32. CDE

Approximately 67% of filtered sodium is actively reabsorbed in the proximal tubule. Although another 25% is reabsorbed in the ascending loop of Henle, it moves passively following active chloride transport. Much of the remaining filtered sodium is reabsorbed from the distal tubule and collecting ducts in exchange for potassium or hydrogen ions. Aldosterone increases sodium reabsorption in the distal parts of the nephron. Increased sodium intake leads to a natriuresis by increasing glomerular filtration rate and natriuretic hormone production, decreasing aldosterone production and by altering Starling forces in peritubular capillaries. The maximum urine concentrating capacity is approximately 400 mosmol/l in preterm infants and is greater than 1200 mosmol/l in normal children.

33. ABD

A false-negative Mantoux test may reflect suppression of the immune system as is the case in high-dose steroid therapy. In miliary tuberculosis the infection is so overwhelming that in effect the child is immunosuppressed. Classically in sarcoidosis, a multisystem chronic granulomatous disorder of unknown aetiology, there is a suppression of cell-mediated immunity leading to false-negative testing.

34. D

When SLE is active the serum complement is depressed. C3 and C4 levels can be used to monitor response to treatment. A poor correlation exists between the clinical manifestations and severity of renal involvement. A biopsy is essential in guiding treatment when renal involvement exists. Neurological involvement is common in SLE. Nearly 50% have neurological problems including: personality disorder, seizures, cardiovascular accidents and a peripheral neuritis (mononeuritis multiplex).

35. **A 1-year-old boy presents in fulminant hepatic failure. The following statements regarding his management are correct:**
    A. if the child is very agitated intravenous sedation should be given.
    B. a partial thromboplastin time (PTT) of greater than 90 seconds is associated with a 100% mortality.
    C. Wilson's disease is a possible diagnosis.
    D. cerebral perfusion pressure (CPP) should be maintained above 50 mmHg.
    E. an emergency liver transplant is indicated if the PTT is greater than 90 seconds.

36. **If two parents are carriers of an autosomal recessive disorder the following statements are true:**
    A. there is a 1 in 3 chance that a child of the carriers will be a carrier.
    B. there is a 1 in 4 chance of having an affected child.
    C. consanguinity increases the risk of having an affected child.
    D. there is a 1 in 4 chance of having a homozygous unaffected child.
    E. Each child will have half its genes in common with its siblings.

37. **The following conditions are associated with bilateral pulmonary hypoplasia:**
    A. preterm prelabour rupture of membranes.
    B. diaphragmatic hernia.
    C. maternal smoking.
    D. myotonic dystrophy.
    E. renal agenesis.

35. BDE

Sedation should never be given to a child in acute hepatic failure unless he/she is ventilated. If sedation is given to an unventilated child, a respiratory arrest can be precipitated resulting in a rise in CO_2 and a worsening of CPP. Sedation can also mask a worsening of a developing encephalopathy. Wilson's disease is not seen in children under 2 years of age. The CPP must be kept above 50 mmHg in order to ensure sufficient blood supply to the brain. It can be calculated from:

$$CPP = \left[(\text{diastolic BP} + \underline{\text{systolic BP} - \text{diastolic BP}}) \right] - ICP$$
$$3$$

(ICP, intracranial pressure). An emergency liver transplant should be considered if any three of the following are present: age <10 years, non-A non-B hepatitis, halothane or other drug-induced hepatitis, jaundice > 7 days before the onset of encephalopathy, PTT > 50 seconds or a serum bilirubin > 300 μmol/l.

36. BCE

In autosomal recessive disorders, homozygous affected individuals will always show signs of the disorder. For this reason the carrier rate for children of heterzygote carriers is 2 in 3 and the chance of being a homozygote unaffected child is 1 in 3.

37. ABDE

The following are associated with pulmonary hypoplasia:

Oligohydramnios	– renal aplasia/severe dysplasia (Potter's syndrome)
	– premature rupture of membranes
	– post-amniocentesis
Compression of lung	– congenital diaphragmatic hernia
	– cystic adenomatoid malformation
	– pleural effusion
	– small chest syndromes
Neuromuscular disease	– spinal muscular atrophy
	– myotonic dystrophy.

38. The following statements regarding coeliac disease are correct:
   A. muscle wasting affects proximal and distal muscle groups cqually.
   B. strict dietary control prevents associated small bowel lymphomas.
   C. the HLA-B8 antigen is present in about 80% of coeliac patients.
   D. dietary restrictions are only necessary in childhood.
   E. a wheat, barley and rye free diet is essential.

39. Methaemoglobinaemia may be caused by:
   A. nitric oxide (NO) therapy.
   B. aniline dyes.
   C. intravenous therapy with glyceryl trinitrate (GTN).
   D. methylene blue.
   E. ascorbic acid.

40. Mastocytosis:
   A. is characterized by aggregates of tissue mast cells in the epidermis.
   B. commonly presents with pruritis.
   C. may be exacerbated by aspirin.
   D. takes the form of a solitary mastocytoma in about 50% of cases.
   E. most commonly takes the form of urticaria pigmentosa.

41. Bloody stools are a recognized clinical feature in children affected by:
   A. verotoxin producing strains of *Escherichia coli*.
   B. *Cryptosporidium*.
   C. *Giardia lamblia*.
   D. cow's milk protein intolerance.
   E. *Ascaris lumbricoides*.

38. CE

Muscle wasting is one of the most consistent features along with failure to thrive, irritability, vomiting and diarrhoea, abdominal distension and offensive stools. Muscle wasting predominantly affects the proximal muscle groups. Strict dietary control does not prevent intestinal malignancies. HLA-B8 antigen is present in about 20% of the general population and in 80% of coeliac patients. Dietary restriction should be life-long. Wheat, rye and probably barley should be avoided.

39. ABC

Oxidation of haemoglobin iron from the ferrous to ferric state produces methaemoglobin, which makes the haemoglobin non-functioning. NO, GTN and other nitrates can produce methaemoglobin, though levels of 2% are definitely safe. Methylene blue and ascorbic acid are used in the treatment of either acquired or inherited methaemoglobinaemia.

40. BCE

Mastocytosis encompasses a spectrum of disorders (mastocytoma, urticaria pigmentosa, diffuse mastocytosis and systemic mastocytosis) with aggregates of mast cells in the dermis. Symptoms result from the release of histamine, which produces a flush, tachycardia, headache, diarrhoea, hypotension, syncope and respiratory distress. It is exacerbated by hot baths, vigorous rubbing, aspirin, codeine, morphine, atropine and polymyxin B. About 10% have a solitary lesion, i.e. mastocytoma.

41. ACD

E. coli O157:H7 (verotoxin producing) is the organism most commonly implicated in haemolytic uraemic syndrome. Other important organisms include shigella and salmonella species. *Cryptosporidium* is a protozoa that causes watery diarrhoea with nausea and abdominal cramps. It may be mild or even asymptomatic but can be a severe problem in immunosuppressed patients, particularly those with AIDS. *Ascaris lumbricoides* is the most prevalent human helminthiasis and most commonly affects preschool and early school-aged children. Infection produces vague abdominal pain, distension and occasionally obstruction in heavy infestations.

42. **The following are abnormal findings in a 7-month-old infant:**
    A. extensor plantar reflex.
    B. Moro reflex.
    C. asymmetrical tonic neck reflex.
    D. obligatory palmar grasp.
    E. crossed adductor spread.

43. **The following statements are true:**
    A. *Neisseria meningitidis* is a gram-negative coccus.
    B. *Haemophilus influenzae* is a gram-positive bacillus.
    C. *Escherichia coli* is a gram-negative bacillus.
    D. *Bordetella pertussis* is a gram-positive bacillus.
    E. *Salmonella* sp. are gram-positive bacilli.

44. **The following are associated with Wilms' tumour:**
    A. cryptorchidism.
    B. hypospadius.
    C. horseshoe kidney.
    D. hemihypertrophy.
    E. aniridia.

42. **BCD**

Plantar reflexes are normally extensor in the newborn and this usually persists for most of the first year of life (found in approximately 75% of normal infants at 12 months of age in one study). The Moro and asymmetrical tonic neck reflexes are abnormal if they persist beyond 6 months of age. The obligatory palmar grasp which is present at birth normally disappears by 2 months of age and is replaced by voluntary grasping from about 4 months of age. Elicitation of the knee tendon jerk at birth usually causes crossed adductor spasm. This normally disappears by 8 months of age.

43. **AC**

Though it is not necessary to have the knowledge of a microbiologist, it is important to know the basic bacterial morphology and classification. We suggest that you learn the following table:

Gram+ve cocci	Gram+ve bacilli	Gram-ve cocci	Gram-ve bacilli
Staph. aureus	*Clostridium sp.*	*N. meningitidis*	*E. coli*
Strep. pyogenes	*Corynebacterium diphtheriae*	*N. gonorrhoeae*	*Salmonella sp.*
Strep. pneumoniae	*Listeria sp.*		*Shigella sp.*
Strep. viridans	*Bacillus anthracis*		*Proteus sp.*
			Klebsiella sp.
			Haemophilus sp.
			Bordetella pertussis
			Pseudomonas sp.

44. **ABCDE**

Children with Wilms' tumour are more likely to have aniridia, hemihypertrophy, genital abnormalities (hypospadius, cryptorchidism) and renal anomalies.

45. **The following drugs induce liver enzyme activity:**
    A. metronidazole.
    B. carbamazepine.
    C. phenytoin.
    D. isoniazid.
    E. chloramphenicol.

46. **The following statements regarding chest disease in children with cystic fibrosis are correct:**
    A. *Pseudomonas aeruginosa* chest infections predominate in children less than 4 years old.
    B. flucloxacillin prophylaxis should be given to all babies with newly diagnosed cystic fibrosis.
    C. *Pseudomonas cepcia* chest infections are associated with a rapid progression of the disease.
    D. reversible airways disease is present in one-third of children with cystic fibrosis.
    E. *Pseudomonas aeruginosa* grown from the nasopharynx is a poor predictor of a lower respiratory tract infection.

47. **The following associations are correct:**
    A. congenital rubella infection – pulmonary stenosis.
    B. maternal diabetes – congenital heart disease.
    C. congenital heart block – seronegative rheumatoid arthritis.
    D. long QT syndrome – atrial tachyarrhythmias.
    E. Noonan's syndrome – pulmonary stenosis.

45. BC

Inducers of liver enzyme activity include:

barbiturates
phenytoin
carbamazepine
alcohol
griseofulvin
rifampicin.

Metronidazole, isoniazid and chloramphenicol are inhibitors of liver enzyme activity.

46. BCD

Staphylococcus aureus infections predominate in younger children with cystic fibrosis. For this reason most units start newborn babies on prophylactic flucloxacillin. *Pseudomonas aeruginosa* when grown from the nasopharynx is highly predictive of lower respiratory tract infection. This is in contrast to *Staph. aureus*, which only has a 50% predictive value. Reversible airways disease in cystic fibrosis may occur in association with acute bronchopulmonary aspergillosis. This needs to be excluded before regular prophylaxis and/or treatment with steroids is commenced if an asthmatic tendency is suspected.

47. ABE

Congenital rubella is associated with both pulmonary stenosis and patent ductus arteriosus (PDA). Infants of diabetics have an increased incidence of congenital heart disease, specifically transposition of the great arteries, ventricular septal defect and PDA. A cardiomyopathy has also been described. Congenital heart block is associated with maternal systemic lupus erythematosus. Long QT syndrome is associated with ventricular tachycardia.

48. **The following conditions typically present with macroscopic haematuria:**
    A. IgA nephropathy.
    B. renal vein thrombosis.
    C. Alport's syndrome.
    D. acute nephritic syndrome.
    E. Fanconi syndrome.

49. **At 5 months of age a normal baby:**
    A. can sit unsupported.
    B. can roll from front to back.
    C. exhibits the Moro reflex.
    D. uses a pincer grip.
    E. has head lag present.

50. **Respiration is stimulated by the following:**
    A. hypercarbia.
    B. hypoxia.
    C. acidosis.
    D. increased barometric pressure.
    E. carbon monoxide inhalation.

51. **Necrotizing enterocolitis (NEC) is associated with:**
    A. congenital heart disease.
    B. Hirschsprung's disease.
    C. maternal diabetes mellitus.
    D. breast feeding.
    E. polycythaemia.

48. ABCD

IgA nephropathy (Berger's nephropathy) presents with recurrent gross haematuria with normal renal function. IgA is deposited in the mesangium. In up to 20% of patients a progressive disease can develop with progressive renal dysfunction. Renal vein thrombosis can be associated with asphyxia, dehydration and sepsis in the newborn and with nephrotic syndrome in older children. It presents with gross haematuria and a mass in the flank. Alport's syndrome is usually an autosomal dominant disorder. It is also associated with sensorineural hearing loss. There is a more severe clinical course in males with most developing end stage renal failure by the second or third decade of life. Acute nephritic syndrome is characterized by haematuria, proteinuria, oedema and hypertension. Fanconi syndrome is characterized by glycosuria, phosphaturia, aminoaciduria and proximal renal tubular acidosis.

49. AB

The important developmental milestones reached at 5 months of age include being able to sit unsupported in a tripod position and being able to roll from back to front. Most babies have lost their Moro reflex by 3 months of age.

50. ABC

Respiration is stimulated primarily by medullary chemoreceptors which respond to hypercarbia. The presence of acidosis exaggerates this response. Oxygen only stimulates respiration if levels are very low, e.g. at high altitude (low barometric pressure). This also becomes more important in chronic lung disease when carbon dioxide levels are chronically raised.

51. ABCE

NEC has many risk factors, including the above. Cyanotic heart disease results in tissue hypoxia. In association with therapeutic interventions such as cardiac catheterization, this hypoxia can contribute to the development of NEC. Maternal diabetes is associated with an increased incidence of NEC. This is due to the increased incidence of birth asphyxia, polycythaemia and hypoglycaemia seen in infants of diabetic mothers. Breast feeding, especially in high-risk infants (intrauterine growth retardation, preterm with respiratory distress syndrome), is probably protective.

52. **The following antineoplastic agents are paired with the side-effects commonly encountered in their usage:**
    A. cyclophosphamide – hepatotoxicity.
    B. cisplatin – ototoxicity.
    C. doxorubicin – cardiomyopathy.
    D. methotrexate – haemorrhagic cystitis.
    E. vincristine – bone marrow suppression.

53. **The following statements regarding an ostium primum atrial septal defect (ASD) are correct:**
    A. ostium primum defects usually occur in the lower part of the atrial septum.
    B. defects usually produce mild symptoms.
    C. an ECG may show left anterior hemiblock.
    D. surgery is rarely indicated since the defect is usually of little haemodynamic significance.
    E. exercise restriction is indicated.

54. **The following conditions cause a rise in the level of alpha-fetoprotein:**
    A. tyrosinaemia.
    B. hepatoblastoma.
    C. neural tube defects.
    D. Down's syndrome.
    E. neuroblastoma.

52. BC

Cyclophosphamide is an alkylating agent used in the treatment of solid tumours and lymphomas. It can cause a haemorrhagic cystitis unless administered in conjunction with the drug MESNA. Cisplatin can cause ototoxicity and for this reason hearing function should be monitored both before and after each course of treatment. Doxorubicin is a cytotoxic antibiotic that may cause a cardiomyopathy. For this reason echocardiographs should be carried out before and after therapy, specifically measuring the cardiac ejection fraction. Methotrexate is an antimetabolite that commonly causes bone marrow suppression. Vincristine is one of the few antineoplastic agents that does not cause myelosuppression.

53. AC

An ostium primum ASD is sometimes called a partial atrioventricular septal defect (AVSD). The defect is in the lower atrial septum near the atrioventricular valves. Clefts in the mitral or tricuspid valve may occur. The defect is usually asymptomatic in childhood but congestive heart failure may develop. Clinical findings are similar to secundum ASD but ECG findings are similar to an AVSD with the presence of a left anterior hemiblock. First-degree atrioventricular block occurs in 50% of cases. Elective surgical repair is performed at 3–4 years of age with closure of the defect and reconstruction of the atrioventricular valves. If necessary, early repair can be performed in those children with heart failure or mitral regurgitation.

54. ABC

In tyrosinaemia plasma levels of alpha-fetoprotein are raised. Diagnosis can be made from characteristic changes in plasma amino acids as well as the presence of succinyl acetone in the urine. Most patients with hepatoblastoma will have raised levels of alpha-fetoprotein. Alpha-fetoprotein may be used as a marker for the efficacy of treatment of hepatoblastomas as well as for the detection of recurrence of disease. Alpha-fetoprotein is measured in pregnancy at around 16 weeks gestation and is raised in the presence of a neural tube defect. When used in conjunction with plasma human chorionic gonadotrophin and oestriol levels, a low alpha-fetoprotein can be used to predict Down's syndrome. Specific diagnostic tests for a neuroblastoma involve measuring levels of catecholamines in the urine. These may include dopa, dopamine, homovanillic acid or vanylmandelic acid.

55. **The following are recognized causes of hydrops fetalis:**
    A. fetal tachycardia.
    B. fetal bradycardia.
    C. rhesus isoimmunization.
    D. ABO incompatibility.
    E. twin to twin transfusion.

56. **ARDS (acute respiratory distress syndrome):**
    A. in childhood carries a low mortality.
    B. by definition has bilateral pulmonary infiltrates on chest X-ray.
    C. may be successfully treated in the acute phase with systemic steroids.
    D. in childhood may be usefully treated with nitric oxide (NO) as an adjuvant.
    E. management involves aggressive ventilation to achieve normal $PaCO_2$.

55. **ABCE**
     Causes of hydrops:

Anaemia (10%)	– twin to twin transfusion
	– fetomaternal transfusion
	– rhesus isoimmunization
	– alpha-thalassaemia (homozygous)
	– glucose-6-phosphate dehydrogenase deficiency (homozygous)
	– Gaucher's disease
Cardiovascular system (20%)	
	– fetal cardiac arrhythmias
	– hypoplastic left heart
	– Ebstein's anomaly
	– myocarditis (coxsackie virus)
	– endocardial fibroelastosis
	– closure of foramen ovale
Chromosomal (10%)	– trisomies
	– triploidy
	– Turner's syndrome
Infection (8%)	– parvovirus B19
	– TORCH infections
	– syphilis
Lung (5%)	– congenital diaphragmatic hernia
	– cystic adenomatoid malformation
Rare	– cystic hygroma
	– congenital nephrosis
	– urinary obstruction
	– fetal malignancies
	– choriocarcinoma
	– meconium peritonitis
	– maternal illness (diabetes, pre-eclampsia).

56. **BD**
     ARDS has a high mortality in both adults and children (40–60%). Figures vary depending on the insult leading to the ARDS. Mortality is higher in the presence of sepsis. Methylprednisolone has been shown to be of benefit in the late fibrotic but not the acute phase. NO decreases pulmonary vascular resistance, decreasing pulmonary artery pressure, and improves $\dot{V}/Q$ mismatch.

57. **The following statements regarding pulmonary stenosis are correct:**
    A. it is characteristically present in Turner's syndrome.
    B. if the pulmonary stenosis is severe there is reversed splitting of the second heart sound.
    C. the second heart sound is loud.
    D. exercise tolerance is always reduced.
    E. the p wave on the ECG is widened.

58. **Mendelian dominant inheritance occurs in the following:**
    A. ABO blood group determination.
    B. Rhesus blood group determination.
    C. neurofibromatosis.
    D. myotonic dystrophy.
    E. Marfan syndrome.

59. **The following statements regarding Ewing's sarcoma are correct:**
    A. the treatment of choice is amputation of the affected limb.
    B. there is an increased incidence of the tumour in children with osteogenesis imperfecta.
    C. pain is rarely a presenting symptom.
    D. the femur is the most common site of tumour occurrence.
    E. 30% of children on presentation have metastatic disease.

60. **In childhood ulcerative colitis:**
    A. the peak age of presentation is 5 years of age.
    B. the risk of colonic carcinoma is greatly increased.
    C. commonly involves small and large intestine.
    D. sulphasalazine is useful in acute exacerbations.
    E. perianal involvement is common.

57. All false

Coarctation of the aorta and a bicuspid aortic valve are found in Turner's syndrome. Pulmonary stenosis is often seen in Noonan's syndrome with dysplastic valves. If the stenosis is severe there is a widely split second sound. Reversed splitting of the second sound is found in aortic stenosis. If pulmonary stenosis is severe, the pulmonary component of the heart sound will be quiet or even inaudible. Pulmonary stenosis may be completely asymptomatic. The p wave on the ECG will be peaked as a result of right atrial hypertrophy.

58. ABCDE

See Question 6, Paper 1.

59. CDE

Amputation is not recommended in children with Ewing's sarcoma as most of the tumours are sensitive to radiotherapy and chemotherapy. There is an increased incidence of osteosarcoma in children with osteogenesis imperfecta. With both osteosarcoma and Ewing's sarcoma the most commonly involved bone is the femur. Ewing's sarcoma metastasizes most frequently to the lungs and bone.

60. B

Although ulcerative colitis may rarely present in children as young as 2 years of age, it is much more likely to present in teenagers. Unlike Crohn's disease it is confined to the large intestine and perianal manifestations are uncommon. First-line treatment for acute exacerbations is with systemic steroids, whereas remission may be prolonged with sulphasalazine. Because of the early age of presentation in children, ulcerative colitis is associated with a greatly increased risk of carcinoma of the colon.

Paper 3

1. **The following statements on Down's syndrome are correct:**
   A. the overall risk of having a child with Down's syndrome, irrespective of maternal age, is 1 in 650 live births.
   B. the risk of having another baby with trisomy 21 after the birth of a child with Down's syndrome is the same as that seen in the general population.
   C. Down's syndrome is due to a 14;21 translocation in 30% of cases.
   D. hyperthyroidism is commonly found in children with Down's syndrome.
   E. 30% of children with Down's syndrome have congenital cardiac defects.

2. **Features of Bartter's syndrome are:**
   A. hypertension.
   B. low urinary chloride.
   C. hyperreninaemia.
   D. hyperaldosteronism.
   E. juxtaglomerular hypoplasia.

3. **The following conditions present with cyanosis in the newborn:**
   A. tricuspid atresia.
   B. Ebstein's anomaly.
   C. atrioventricular septal defect (AVSD).
   D. tetralogy of Fallot.
   E. transient myocardial ischaemia.

1. **AE**
   The risk of having a child with Down's syndrome increases with maternal age, reaching 1 in 40 in women over the age of 44 years. After having had one child with Down's syndrome the risk of having another child with trisomy 21 is 1 in 200. In about 5% of cases, Down's syndrome can be shown to be due to a translocation. In less than half these cases one of the parents can be shown to be carrying a balanced version of the translocation. Hypothyroidism is commonly seen in children with Down's syndrome and thyroid function tests should be performed annually.

2. **CD**
   Bartter's syndrome presents with failure to thrive, muscle weakness, polyuria and normal blood pressure. Biochemical features include hypokalaemia (usually < 2.5 mmol/l), hypo-chloridaemia, metabolic alkalosis, high urinary chloride and potassium. Hyperreninaemia, hyperaldosteronism and raised prostaglandin E_2 may also be present. Bartter's syndrome can be inherited as an autosomal condition. The syndrome is thought to be due to a defect in chloride reabsorption in the ascending limb of the loop of Henle.

3. **ABD**
   Cardiac conditions that present with cyanosis in neonates include:

   > transposition of the great arteries (TGA)
   > pulmonary atresia
   > severe pulmonary stenosis
   > severe tetralogy of Fallot
   > tricuspid atresia
   > Ebstein's anomaly
   > total anomalous pulmonary venous drainage (TAPVD)
   > hypoplastic left heart
   > truncus arteriosus.

   Babies with AVSD usually become symptomatic after the first 2 weeks of life with symptoms and signs of congestive cardiac failure. Transient myocardial ischaemia is often a feature of perinatal asphyxia. It may cause varying degrees of congestive cardiac failure or may only be evident as temporary ECG changes.

4. **A 3-month-old-girl who had previously been well presents in outpatients. She has no physical signs apart from being irritable and the fact that she seems to have regressed developmentally. The following are possible diagnoses:**
   A. Menkes syndrome.
   B. congenital hypothyroidism.
   C. maple syrup urine disease.
   D. Tay-Sachs' disease.
   E. hydrocephalus.

5. **The following statements are true:**
   A. the precursor of all steroid hormones is cholesterol.
   B. prednisolone is a more potent glucocorticoid than dexamethasone.
   C. fludrocortisone has potent mineralocorticoid activity.
   D. dexamethasone has potent mineralocorticoid activity.
   E. cortisol has glucocorticoid and mineralocorticoid activity.

6. **The following agents are paired with their appropriate mechanism of action:**
   A. vigabatrin   –   GABA agonist.
   B. lamotrigine   –   inhibition of glutamate release.
   C. methyldopa   –   beta-adrenergic receptor agonist.
   D. baclofen   –   GABA beta receptor agonist.
   E. acetazolamide   –   carbonic anhydrase inhibitor.

4. BDE

Developmental regression can be due to a wide variety of conditions. Menkes syndrome is a sex-linked recessive disease that results from an abnormality of copper metabolism. Developmental retardation becomes apparent during the first few months of life. Scalp hair is initially normal but becomes sparse and brittle. In congenital hypothyroidism the infant may initially appear normal. Developmental regression will almost always have started by 3 months. In maple syrup urine disease, affected infants are normal at birth but become unwell during the first week of life with poor feeding, hypoglycaemia and coma. In Tay-Sachs' disease an infant who has previously been well becomes apathetic and acquires an exaggerated startle reflex. The condition is due to hexosaminidase A deficiency. Characteristically a cherry-red spot is visible on the macula. Slow-developing hydrocephalus may also present with developmental regression.

5. ACE

Dexamethasone has no mineralocorticoid activity but has approximately five times the glucocorticoid activity of prednisolone. Fludrocortisone has a powerful mineralocorticoid effect and some glucocorticoid activity. Cortisol has relatively weak glucocorticoid and mineralocorticoid effects.

6. BDE

Vigabatrin is a recently developed anti-epileptic agent. It acts by selectively and irreversibly inhibiting the enzyme GABA transaminase. This increases the levels of GABA which is the major inhibitory neurotransmitter in the brain. Lamotrigine is another anti-epileptic agent and acts on voltage-sensitive sodium channels. This stabilizes neuronal membranes and glutamate release is inhibited. Glutamate is thought to have a key excitatory role in the generation of epileptic seizures. Methyldopa is a centrally acting antihypertensive agent. It is metabolized to alpha-methyladrenaline and stimulates central inhibitory alpha-adrenergic receptors. Baclofen stimulates GABA beta receptors, which inhibit glutamate and aspartate release thus depressing synaptic transmission and relieving spasticity of voluntary muscles.

7. **The following features make a diagnosis of ulcerative colitis more likely than one of Crohn's disease:**
   A. perianal lesions.
   B. crypt abscesses on biopsy.
   C. granulomata.
   D. pyoderma gangrenosum.
   E. presence of a fistula.

8. **According to the 1989 Children Act the following principles and provisions are applicable if child abuse is suspected:**
   A. an emergency protection order lasts for 8 days.
   B. a child assessment order allows a child to be taken into local authority care.
   C. the welfare of the child is paramount.
   D. the length of an emergency protection order cannot be extended.
   E. a child assessment order can be granted by a local authority.

9. **The following are true regarding cardiovascular changes at around birth:**
   A. the umbilical vein closes before the umbilical arteries.
   B. the umbilical arteries are attached to the aorta.
   C. closure of the ductus arteriosus can be delayed by maternal ingestion of aspirin.
   D. the foramen ovale is permanently closed by 6 weeks.
   E. fetal oxygen levels are at 4 kPa (30 mmHg).

10. **Obstructive sleep apnoea (OSA) in children:**
   A. is more pronounced in rapid eye movement (REM) sleep.
   B. results in reduced synthesis of neurotransmitters.
   C. causes bradycardia and other arrhythmias.
   D. does not lead to permanent changes of pulmonary vasculature.
   E. treatment of choice is adenoidectomy.

7. BD

Perianal lesions and the development of a fistula are highly suggestive of Crohn's disease. Histological features of ulcerative colitis include mucosal disease with crypt abscesses, decreased goblet cells and an infiltration of polymorphs. Granulomata are not a feature of ulcerative colitis but pyoderma gangrenosum does occasionally develop.

8. AC

In the 1989 Children Act it is stated that the welfare of the child is paramount. An emergency protection order allows a child to be taken into care and lasts for 8 days. It may be extended at the discretion of the court for a further 7 days. After 3 days the parent or the child may challenge the order. A child assessment order allows medical or psychiatric examination to be carried out. A full court order is necessary. If the parents or carers do not cooperate, the assessment order may be converted to an emergency protection order.

9. E

The umbilical arteries are attached to the common iliac arteries. Although the exact mechanism by which the ductus arteriosus closes is not known, prostaglandin E_2 is involved in maintenance of the patency of the duct. In theory maternal aspirin ingestion may cause premature closure of the duct although this is controversial. The foramen ovale is functionally open at 6 weeks. In most infants it is permanently closed by 3 months of age, although in up to 25% of individuals it is possible to pass a probe between the unfused flaps in later life.

10. ABC

There are two factors that are important in the development of obstructive sleep apnoea (OSA): firstly, tonsil and adenoid hypertrophy; and secondly the loss of tone in the tongue and pharyngeal wall in sleep. The latter is more pronounced in REM sleep. OSA causes a reduction in neurotransmitter levels, which together with sleep fragmentation accounts for daytime somnolence. A range of vagally mediated arrhythmias, most commonly bradycardia, result from hypoxia. Permanent changes in the pulmonary arterial vasculature and cor pulmonale are well described. Treatment of choice is adeno-tonsillectomy because adenoidectomy alone does not consistently cure OSA.

11. **Pulmonary plethora on a chest X-ray is seen in:**
    A. tetralogy of Fallot.
    B. atrial septal defect (ASD).
    C. partial anomalous pulmonary venous drainage (PAPVD).
    D. tricuspid atresia.
    E. Ebstein's anomaly.

12. **The following statements regarding the treatment of malaria are correct:**
    A. prophylaxis is not necessary in breast-fed babies if the mother is taking chloroquine regularly.
    B. chloroquine alone is sufficient in the treatment of *Plasmodium vivax.*
    C. primaquine treatment is necessary in order to clear parasites from the liver in *Plasmodium malariae* infection.
    D. prophylaxis should continue for 3 months after the return of a child from an area where malaria is endemic.
    E. if the species of infecting malaria is not known, chloroquine is the treatment of choice.

13. **The following statements are correct:**
    A. following the introduction of the MMR vaccine it is no longer necessary to vaccinate against rubella in 10 to 14-year-old girls.
    B. the Hib vaccine is a capsular conjugated polysaccharide.
    C. immunoglobulin must not be given with the MMR vaccine.
    D. hepatitis B vaccine is contraindicated in pregnancy.
    E. the mumps component of the MMR is a live vaccine.

11. **BC**

    Pulmonary vascular markings should be assessed on the chest X-ray of any child suspected of having a congenital heart defect. Increased markings are seen when there is increased flow through the pulmonary vasculature as in a left to right shunt. Increased markings may also be seen when there is outflow obstruction to the left side of the heart such as with total anomalous pulmonary venous drainage and coarctation of the aorta.

12. **All false**

    Although antimalarials are excreted in breast milk, the amounts present are too variable to give reliable protection. A combination of chloroquine and proguanil (dose adjusted for age or weight) is recommended. In order to eliminate *P. vivax* or *P. ovale* from the liver a course of primaquine for up to 21 days is essential. *P. malariae* is cleared by a course of chloroquine by itself. Prophylaxis should start 1 week before travelling into an area where malaria is endemic and continue for 4 weeks after returning. If the species of malaria is not known in a child presenting with what appears to be malaria, treatment should be with quinine, halofantrine or mefloquine as if one was treating *P. falciparum.*

13. **BCE**

    From September 1994 the MR vaccine should be given to all children aged 5–16 years in school. There are two brands of Hib vaccines, both of which are capsular conjugated polysaccharide vaccines. They are not interchangeable since they are conjugated with different proteins. Immunoglobulin must not be given with the MMR since the immune response to rubella and mumps may be inhibited. Live vaccines are not routinely given to pregnant women but if there is a significant risk of exposure the benefits of vaccination may outweigh the risks to the fetus. Since the hepatitis B vaccine contains inactivated virus surface antigen (HBsAg) it can be given in pregnancy. All parts of the MMR are live.

14. **The following statements regarding Alagille syndrome are correct:**
    A. posterior embryotoxon is pathognomonic of the syndrome.
    B. extrahepatic biliary atresia is a feature.
    C. cholesterol levels are usually raised.
    D. aortic stenosis is found in most cases.
    E. renal abnormalities are present in most cases.

15. **The following conditions can produce a pruritic rash:**
    A. granuloma annulare.
    B. eczema.
    C. lichen planus.
    D. dermatitis herpetiformis.
    E. pityriasis rosea.

16. **The following statements are correct:**
    A. the perinatal mortality rate is the number of deaths in the first 28 days of life per 1000 live births per annum.
    B. the prevalence rate of a given condition is the proportion of a defined population having a condition at any one time.
    C. case control studies are useful when investigating rare diseases.
    D. cross-sectional studies give an estimate of the incidence of a given disease.
    E. cross-sectional studies can provide information as to the temporal relationship between a causative agent and a disease.

14. **CE**

Alagille syndrome is associated with intrahepatic biliary hypoplasia. It is usually inherited as an autosomal dominant condition with variable expression, although in some cases Alagille syndrome can be inherited in an autosomal recessive manner. Posterior embryotoxon is accumulated material on the inner aspect of the cornea near the junction with the iris. Although typically it is present in Alagille syndrome it is also present in up to 10% of the normal population. Posterior embryotoxon can only be seen on slit lamp examination. Cholesterol and triglyceride levels are raised in almost all cases. Xanthelasma are rare in children less than 2 years old with the condition but are commonly present after puberty. Peripheral pulmonary artery stenosis is typically present. The renal abnormality is usually a tubulointerstitial nephropathy.

15. **BCDE**

Granulomare annulare is a benign, non-pruritic condition that presents with erythematous, firm nodules which coalesce to form ring-shaped lesions. Lichen planus produces an intensely pruritic rash that shows the Koebner phenomenon in that scratching produces new lesions. Dermatitis herpetiformis produces erythematous, pruritic papules and vesicles. It is associated with coeliac disease. Pityriasis rosea is characteristically preceded by a herald patch 5–10 days before the eruption of the rash. Lesions are typically oval, slightly raised and are pink/brown in colour. The rash may be severely pruritic or asymptomatic.

16. **BC**

The perinatal mortality rate is the number of stillbirths and deaths after 24 weeks gestation in the first week of life per 1000 live births. The definition quoted in the question is the neonatal mortality rate. The prevalence rate is a useful measure when a condition being investigated is relatively stable. However, it will underestimate the true number of affected individuals because of deaths. Cross-sectional studies estimate the prevalence of a condition. Cohort or case control studies need to be carried out if a temporal relationship between a disease and a causative agent is to be investigated.

17. **A 1-year-old child presents with a suspected neuroblastoma. The following statements are correct:**
    A. a neuroblastoma may spontaneously regress.
    B. a bone marrow aspirate should be carried out on all children suspected of having a neuroblastoma.
    C. diarrhoea is a recognized presenting symptom.
    D. calcification is rarely present in the tumour.
    E. neuroblastomas are rarely radiosensitive.

18. **A term newborn infant is noticed to be hypotonic. The following are possible causes:**
    A. Turner's syndrome.
    B. Kugelberg-Welander disease.
    C. cephalhaematoma.
    D. Prader-Willi syndrome.
    E. galactosaemia.

19. **Target cells appear in the peripheral blood film in the following conditions:**
    A. chronic liver disease.
    B. beta-thalassaemia.
    C. vitamin B_{12} deficiency.
    D. haemoglobin C disease.
    E. sickle cell disease.

17. **ABC**

Spontaneous regression of neuroblastoma tumours may occur, especially in infants with stage I or IV disease. In order to stage the tumour a bone marrow aspirate must be carried out in all children with the disease. In severe cases the entire bone marrow can be replaced by tumour, resulting in pancytopenia. Rarely, severe diarrhoea can occur as the result of the production of vasoactive intestinal peptide by the tumour. This stops once the tumour is removed. Calcification is present in 80% of tumours although a computed tomographic scan is sometimes required for the calcification to be seen. Most neuroblastoma tumours are radiosensitive although chemotherapy is used in widely disseminated disease.

18. **DE**

Causes of neonatal hypotonia can be classified anatomically:

systemic: sepsis, trisomies, metabolic disease, e.g. galactosaemia, drugs, etc.
brain: hypoxic ischaemic encephalopathy, intracranial haemorrhage, malformations
spinal cord: birth trauma, spina bifida, tumour
anterior horn cell: spinal muscular atrophy
neuromuscular junction: neonatal myasthenia gravis
muscle: congenital myopathies, benign congenital hypotonia.

19. **ABDE**

Target-shaped red blood cells with normal haemoglobin content are present in homozygous haemoglobin C disease. This is a relatively benign condition that results in splenomegaly and red blood cells with increased osmotic fragility. The most common cause of target cells is liver disease. Hypochromic target cells appear in the thalassaemias and in sickle cell disease.

20. **Post-haemorrhagic hydrocephalus following intraventricular haemorrhage (IVH) in preterm infants:**
    A. is often due to blockage of the outflow of the 4th ventricle.
    B. never results in microcephaly.
    C. is always associated with moderate to severe neurodevelopmental impairment.
    D. may be treated with acetazolamide.
    E. rarely undergoes spontaneous remission.

21. **In cystic fibrosis:**
    A. acute sinusitis is common.
    B. 30% of patients have gastrointestinal symptoms.
    C. haemolytic anaemia may develop.
    D. vitamin E deficiency occurs.
    E. most males have obliterated or atretic vas deferens.

22. **Causes of pancreatitis in childhood include:**
    A. prednisolone.
    B. azathioprine.
    C. systemic lupus erythematosis (SLE).
    D. hyperlipidaemia.
    E. hypocalcaemia.

23. **The following milk feeds are lactose free:**
    A. Formula S.
    B. Wysoy.
    C. Pregestemil.
    D. SMA gold cap.
    E. Cow and Gate premium.

20. BD

Organization of blood clot following a large intraventricular haemorrhage often results in scarring of the outflow from the 4th ventricle (foraminae of Magendie and Luschke) or at the arachnoid villi. The subsequent obstruction of cerebrospinal fluid (CSF) outflow leads to ventricular dilatation which may result in hydrocephalus. About 25% of cases of post-haemorrhagic ventricular dilatation (PHVD) undergo spontaneous remission. Acetazolamide may help by reducing the rate of CSF production. Subsequent cerebral atrophy may be severe enough for microcephaly to occur. Following PHVD approximately 40–60% of children have a major handicap.

21. CDE

Blocked nasal passages and rhinitis are common in cystic fibrosis as a result of nasal polyps and inflamed mucosa. Paranasal sinuses are virtually opacified on X-ray but acute sinusitis is infrequent. About 85% have gastrointestinal symptoms. Haemolytic anaemia is well described and can result from vitamin E deficiency. Deficiencies of all fat-soluble vitamins (A, D, E and K) may occur. The vas deferens, epididymis and seminal vesicles are obliterated or atretic.

22. ABCD

Most cases of pancreatitis occur after the age of 10 years. About 20% of cases are idiopathic. Causes include: drugs (diuretics, prednisolone, alcohol, azathioprine), trauma, infections (mumps, hepatitis A and B, rubella, coxsackie A, influenza and parainfluenza), Reyes syndrome, SLE, hyperlipidaemia types I, IV and V and hypercalcaemia.

23. ABC

Lactase seems to be the most vulnerable brush border enzyme. For this reason activity can be reduced after insults to the mucosal lining of the gastrointestinal tract. This can happen after acute gastroenteritis, coeliac disease in relapse, after hypoxic episodes and in protein energy malnutrition. Recovery is the general rule in such cases after treatment with lactose-free milks. Formula S is a soya-based milk, as is Wysoy. Pregestemil is a whole-protein-free milk and contains medium chain triglycerides for ease of absorption.

24. The following statements are true:
   A. alkaline phosphatase levels are raised in hypophosphatasia.
   B. tetany is present in familial hypophosphataemia.
   C. treatment of familial hypophosphataemia requires vitamin D_2 doses of 2000 IU/kg/24 hours.
   D. all children with rickets have osteomalacia.
   E. rickets can be present in proximal tubular acidosis.

25. Nitric oxide (NO):
   A. is produced endogenously in epithelial cells.
   B. when inhaled 20–40% is absorbed into the bloodstream to form methaemoglobin.
   C. therapy producing a methaemoglobin level of 10% is considered insignificant.
   D. can produce prolonged bleeding time.
   E. is an endogenous neurotransmitter.

26. Respiratory syncytial virus (RSV):
   A. is the most common cause of pneumonia in the 1st year of life.
   B. invariably causes wheezing during acute bronchiolitis.
   C. infection can be confirmed by a viral immunofluorescent technique in over 90% of infected cases.
   D. is the organism responsible for obliterative bronchiolitis.
   E. acute bronchiolitis is associated with subsequent episodes of cough and wheeze in over 50% of cases.

27. The following statements are true:
   A. adrenaline has alpha-adrenergic activity only.
   B. dopamine has both alpha- and beta-adrenergic activity.
   C. isoprenaline acts by alpha-adrenergic stimulation.
   D. alpha-adrenergic stimulation results in vasodilatation.
   E. salbutamol is a β_2 agonist.

24. CDE

Hypophosphatasia resembles rickets on X-ray and is characterized by low serum alkaline phosphatase levels. Familial hypophosphataemia or vitamin D resistant rickets is an X-linked dominant condition that requires phosphate supplements together with vitamin D analogues for adequate bone healing to occur. Rickets occurs in proximal tubular acidosis as a result of phosphate loss and the acidosis impairing the conversion of $25(OH)D$ to $1,25(OH)_2D$.

25. DE

NO is produced in the vascular endothelium, macrophages and some neuronal cells within the brain. Eighty to ninety per cent of inhaled NO is absorbed into the blood to form methaemoglobin. Fatal methaemoglobinaemia with chronic NO use >10 ppm in humans has to be reported. NO has many roles in addition to that of modulation of vascular tone, including in the host defence system, as a neurotransmitter and in intestinal motility. NO prevents clot formation by preventing platelet aggregation and bleeding time may be prolonged although this is rarely of clinical significance.

26. ACE

RSV is the most common cause of pneumonia in infancy. Babies with RSV acute bronchiolitis typically have tachypnoea, intercostal recession and hyperinflation and on auscultation of the chest, fine crackles with or without wheeze. Diagnosis of RSV infection can be rapidly confirmed by detection of viral antigens in nasal secretion by immunofluorescent techniques. This is over 90% sensitive and specific compared with tissue culture techniques. Follow-up studies on babies admitted to hospital with acute bronchiolitis suggest that a large number (50–80%) subsequently develop recurrent episodes of coughing and wheezing. The organism responsible for obliterative bronchiolitis is usually adenovirus.

27. BE

Adrenaline has alpha- and beta-adrenergic activity. Dopamine has dopaminergic activity at low doses and alpha- and beta-adrenergic activity at higher doses. Isoprenaline is a nonspecific beta agonist, whereas salbutamol is a β_2 agonist. Alpha-adrenergic stimulation leads to vasoconstriction.

28. A 1-year-old girl presents in clinic whose father has been shown to have *Mycobacterium tuberculosis* present in his sputum. The child's chest X-ray is normal and she has not had the BCG vaccination. A Mantoux test is negative. The following statements regarding further management are correct:
    A. BCG vaccination should be given immediately.
    B. if a Mantoux test is negative there is no need for tuberculosis chemoprophylaxis.
    C. the chemoprophylactic agent of choice is rifampicin.
    D. chemoprophylaxis should continue for 1 year.
    E. BCG should be given if a Mantoux test in 6 months time is negative.

29. The following conditions require surgical management in the newborn period:
    A. phimosis.
    B. cavernous haemangioma.
    C. Hirschsprung's disease.
    D. umbilical hernia.
    E. tongue tie.

28. E

According to the British Thoracic Society guidelines published in 1994, children under the age of 2 years who have not had a BCG and are a close contact of a sputum-positive adult should have chemoprophylaxis irrespective of tuberculin status. Isoniazid is the agent of choice and treatment should continue for 6 months, after which time a repeat Mantoux test should be carried out. If this is still negative the BCG vaccination should be given.

29. C

The foreskin is non-retractile in the immediate newborn period and traumatic forced retraction may predispose to later phimosis by causing scarring. Cavernous haemangiomas (strawberry naevi) are common and only very rarely require treatment with systemic steroids or surgery if they interfere with vision or ability to feed. Most enlarge over the next few months and then subsequently regress. Hirschsprung's disease presenting in the neonatal period requires surgical management with either resection of the aganglionic segment or formation of a colostomy proximal to the affected segment. Surgery may be delayed if the gut can be kept decompressed by regular rectal washouts or rectal stimulation. Umbilical hernias usually resolve by about 2 years of age and only require surgery for cosmetic reasons if they persist for longer. Tongue tie or short frenulum only requires surgical treatment in the most extreme cases and otherwise parental reassurance is all that is required.

30. **The following statements regarding the external ocular muscles of the eye and their nerve supplies are correct:**
    A. the lateral rectus is almost solely responsible for adduction of the eye.
    B. the inferior oblique and the superior rectus are responsible for upward movement of the eye.
    C. the abducens nerve (VI) supplies the lateral rectus muscle.
    D. the oculomotor nerve (III) may be damaged by a cavernous sinus thrombosis.
    E. abducens nerve palsy may occur in raised intracranial pressure.

31. **Gynaecomastia can be found in the following conditions:**
    A. two-thirds of pubescent boys.
    B. hypothyroidism.
    C. Klinefelter syndrome.
    D. liver cirrhosis.
    E. ketoconazole therapy.

30. BCDE

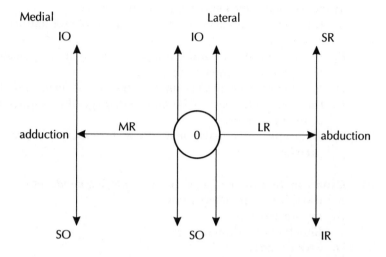

[Inferior Oblique (IO), Superior Rectus (SR), Medial Rectus (MR), Superior Oblique (SO), Inferior Rectus (IR)]
The lateral rectus (LR) muscle is supplied by the sixth cranial nerve (abducens nerve), and the superior oblique (SO) muscle by the fourth cranial nerve (trochlear nerve). All other muscles are supplied by the third cranial nerve (oculomotor nerve). A cavernous sinus thrombosis may affect the IIIrd, IVth and VIth cranial nerves. Pressure on the VIth cranial nerve, in conditions where raised intracranial pressure is present, can produce a false localizing sign due to paralysis of the lateral rectus muscle.

31. ABCDE

Gynaecomastia can be a transient phenomenon in up to two-thirds of male adolescents. This is associated with a decreased testosterone to oestriol levels. Gynaecomastia in liver cirrhosis occurs as a result of decreased metabolism of oestrogens. Ketoconazole therapy directly inhibits testosterone synthesis resulting in gynaecomastia. Gynaecomastia occurs in hypo- and hyperthyroidism. The mechanism behind this is not known.

32. **The following statements regarding the diagnosis and management of iritis are correct:**
    A. the pupil of the affected eye will be dilated and irregular.
    B. if the eye is painful a diagnosis of iritis is unlikely.
    C. the most common systemic association with iritis in children is with juvenile rheumatoid arthritis.
    D. atropine can be used in therapy.
    E. retinal detachment is a recognized complication.

33. **The following statements regarding a patent ductus arteriosus (PDA) are correct:**
    A. in the presence of a large shunt across the PDA the chest X-ray findings include cardiomegaly and increased pulmonary vascular markings.
    B. a continuous murmur is diagnostic.
    C. subacute bacterial endocarditis (SBE) prophylaxis is not indicated.
    D. PDA accounts for about 5–10% of all congenital heart disease in term infants.
    E. during fetal life the ductus carries oxygenated blood in a right to left shunt.

34. **Sickle cell anaemia:**
    A. results from the substitution of leucine for valine on the beta-haemoglobin chain.
    B. antenatal diagnosis is not yet possible.
    C. symptoms are rare before 6 months of age.
    D. haemoglobin A2 is present in normal amounts.
    E. rapid solubility tests provide the most accurate diagnosis.

32. **CDE**

Inflammation of the anterior part of the uveal tract can present either as iritis or cyclitis (ciliary body inflammation). Iritis presents with photophobia, pain, blurred vision and a small and irregular pupil. Iritis is most commonly associated with juvenile rheumatoid arthritis although it is also seen in toxoplasmosis, histoplasmosis, sarcoidosis, tuberculosis, mumps, measles and herpes simplex infection. A cycloplegic such as atropine is given to dilate the pupil and relieve iris spasm. Topical corticosteroids are also indicated as long as a viral infection is not thought to be present. Complications such as retinal detachment and glaucoma are sometimes seen.

33. **ADE**

Small PDAs are asymptomatic. The diameter and length of the PDA and pulmonary vascular resistance determine the extent of the shunt across the heart. There are many causes of continuous murmurs. These include: arteriovenous fistulas, a venous hum, collaterals in patients with coarctation of the aorta or tetralogy of Fallot, ventricular septal defect with aortic regurgitation, absent pulmonary valve syndrome, and truncus arteriosus. The exact nature and position of the murmur of a PDA is described as continuous machinery, grade 1–4/6 maximum at upper left sternal border or infraclavicular area.

34. **CD**

Homozygous sickle cell disease results from a single gene mutation for the synthesis of beta-globin chains. Valine occurs instead of glutamine in the 6 position. DNA analysis of fetal tissue makes antenatal diagnosis possible after chorionic villous biopsy. The predominance of fetal haemoglobin in the first few months of life means that sickle cell disease rarely causes problems before 4–6 months of age. The proportion of fetal haemoglobin is increased in children with homozygous sickle cell disease (5–15%), whereas the proportion of haemoglobin A2 remains normal (2–3%). The most reliable diagnostic test is haemoglobin electrophoresis, which shows an absence of haemoglobin A and preponderance of haemoglobin S.

35. The following statements are correct:
A. the foregut gives rise to the duodenum and jejunum.
B. the ascending colon is derived from the hindgut.
C. if the urorectal septum fails to develop, a fistula may occur between the rectum and bladder.
D. the glomerulus is derived from the mesonephron.
E. the cloaca only gives rise to the bladder.

36. If one carries out a Valsalva manoeuvre against a closed glottis the following will occur:
A. a rise in intrathoracic pressure.
B. a rise in left ventricular output.
C. a rise in blood pressure.
D. a fall in heart rate.
E. a fall in right ventricular output.

37. The following vaccines contain live attenuated viruses:
A. measles, mumps and rubella (MMR).
B. yellow fever.
C. rubella.
D. hepatitis B.
E. poliomyelitis (sabin).

38. In Gilbert's syndrome:
A. diagnosis is usually made in the first year of life.
B. asymptomatic jaundice is the usual mode of presentation.
C. a conjugated hyperbilirubinaemia occurs.
D. liver enzymes are usually mildly elevated with evidence of haemolysis.
E. the underlying defect is defective or absent uridine diphosphate glucuronyl transferase (UDPGT) activity.

35. C

The foregut gives rise to the larynx, pharynx, oesophagus, stomach and duodenum. The midgut gives rise to the duodenum and gut through to the proximal two-thirds of the transverse colon. The hindgut gives rise to the distal third of the colon, rectum and upper anal canal. The kidney is derived from the metanephros (glomeruli, proximal and distal tubules). The lower part of the mesonephric (Wolffian) duct gives rise to the ureteric bud, which will constitute the collecting system.

36. AE

Owing to increased intrathoracic pressure, there is a fall in right ventricular output because of decreased venous return to the heart. There is therefore a fall in left ventricular output and a concomitant fall in blood pressure.

37. ABCE

Live vaccines are polio (oral or sabin), measles, mumps, rubella, yellow fever and BCG.

38. B

The diagnosis of Gilbert's syndrome, a chronic, mild, variable unconjugated hyperbilirubinaemia without significant haemolysis or abnormality of liver enzymes, is rarely made with confidence before the age of 10 years. The pathogenesis is undetermined but impaired hepatic uptake of bilirubin and deficient glucuronyl transferase activity is implicated. The complete absence of the enzyme bilirubin uridine diphosphate glucuronyl transferase (UDPGT) occurs in the autosomal recessive condition Crigler-Najjar syndrome type I.

39. **The following associations regarding the inheritance of conditions that affect drug metabolism are correct:**
    A. rapid acetylator status   – autosomal recessive.
    B. suxamethonium sensitivity   – autosomal recessive.
    C. glucose-6-phosphate dehydro-
      genase (G6PD) deficiency   – X-linked dominant.
    D. acute intermittent porphyria   – autosomal dominant.
    E. malignant hyperthermia   – autosomal recessive.

40. **A mother presents to an antenatal clinic in the UK who is 28 weeks pregnant. She is found to be HIV positive. The following statements are correct:**
    A. the risk of her transmitting the infection to her baby is greater than 50%.
    B. the presence of p24 antigenaemia in the mother increases the risk of vertical transmission.
    C. breast feeding the infant is recommended.
    D. zidovudine should be given to the mother in the antenatal period.
    E. zidovudine should not be given to the infant until the results of an HIV test are known.

41. **Concerning immunoglobulin antibody molecules, the following statements are true:**
    A. the Fc portion binds antigen.
    B. there are four light chains and four heavy chains.
    C. complement binds to the Fab portion.
    D. two different types of light chain occur.
    E. immunoglobulin G and immunoglobulin M are involved in complement fixation.

39. BD

About 40% of Caucasians have rapid acetylator status with increased hepatic acetylase activity towards drugs such as isoniazid, hydralazine and sulphonamides. Rapid acetylation has an autosomal dominant mode of inheritance. Several types of abnormal plasma pseudocholinesterases account for suxamethonium sensitivity. Drugs that can precipitate haemolysis in children with G6PD include: nitrofurantoin, primaquine, sulphonamides and salicylates. Drugs that can precipitate an attack of porphyria include: carbamazepine, chloroquine, phenytoin and rifampicin. Malignant hyperthermia, an autosomal dominant condition, is a potentially fatal complication of general anaesthetic with halothane, methoxyflurane or succinylcholine. Dantrolene may be used in treatment.

40. BD

The risk of mother to child transmission of HIV ranges from 15 to 35%. The lower figure is that reported in Europe. Vertical transmission depends on several factors. Viral load seems to be important and the presence of p24 antigen, which indicates active infection, has been shown to increase transmission rates. Breast feeding is not recommended in developed countries as the virus has been shown to be present in breast milk. In developing countries, the risks of bottle feeding infants probably outweigh the benefits seen by not breast feeding so the recommendations are different. It has been shown that giving antenatal and intrapartum zidovudine to pregnant women before 34 weeks gestation, who have not been previously treated with antiviral drugs, who have CD4 counts of over 200 per mm^3 and who are not breast feeding, reduces the transmission rate by about two-thirds. Zidovudine should also be given to the infant for 6 weeks before any HIV test results are known.

41. DE

Two light chains and two heavy chains form the immunoglobulin molecule. The Fab portion is involved in antigen recognition and binding. The Fc portion binds macrophages and complement. Two types of light chain (k and l) and eight types of heavy chain occur.

42. The following statements regarding extrahepatic biliary atresia (EHBA) are correct:
A. the incidence of EHBA is 1 in 14 000 live births.
B. pigmented stools exclude a diagnosis of EHBA.
C. definitive diagnosis of EHBA is made from liver biopsy.
D. treatment of choice is the Kasai operation.
E. prognosis for clearing the jaundice is greater than 70% if diagnosis and treatment are made before 70 days of age.

43. William's syndrome is associated with:
A. failure to thrive.
B. hyperacusis.
C. learning difficulties.
D. hypocalcaemia.
E. an autosomal dominant mode of inheritance.

44. For a diagnostic test, the following statements are correct:
A. the sensitivity is the proportion of true positives correctly identified by the test.
B. the specificity is the proportion of false positives.
C. sensitivity and specificity are affected by the prevalence.
D. the positive predictive value is the proportion of patients with a positive test correctly diagnosed.
E. the negative predictive value is the proportion of patients with a positive test incorrectly diagnosed.

42. AD

Pigmented stools have been reported in up to 30% of infants with EHBA. Even experienced histopathologists can only diagnose or exclude bilary duct obstruction in 77% of cases. Definitive diagnosis can only be made on laparotomy. The treatment of choice is the Kasai operation (hepatic portoenterostomy). If diagnosis and treatment are made before 60 days, infants have a 70–90% chance of clearing their jaundice. The success rate falls to 30–60% if the diagnosis is not made until 61–70 days.

43. BC

William's syndrome occurs sporadically in virtually all known cases. Children with the condition have typical elfin-like features with a small mandible, peg-like teeth and a prominent philtrum. They usually have learning difficulties and have a 'cocktail party' personality. Hypercalcaemia can be seen, which can lead to nephrocalcinosis. The typical heart lesion seen with this condition is supravalvular aortic stenosis although peripheral pulmonary stenosis and aortic hypoplasia are also seen.

44. AD

Sensitivity, specificity, positive predictive value (PPV) and negative predictive value (NPV) are used to assess the accuracy of a diagnostic test. Sensitivity is the proportion of true positives correctly identified by the test. Specificity is the proportion of true negatives correctly identified by the test. Sensitivity and specificity are not affected by the prevalence of the condition being tested for. The accuracy of the test may be assessed in a more clinically useful way by considering the PPV and the NPV. The proportion of patients with a positive test who are correctly diagnosed is called PPV, whereas the proportion of patients with a negative test correctly diagnosed is the NPV. This can be summarized using the table below:

	Disease		
	Present	Absent	Total
Test			
Positive	a	b	a + b
Negative	c	d	c + d
Total	a + c	b + d	n

Sensitivity=a/(a+c).   PPV=a/(a+b).
Specificity=d/(b+d).   NPV=d/(c+d).

45. **In haemolytic anaemias:**
    A. hereditary spherocytosis (HS) is the most common cause in Northern Europeans.
    B. HS is inherited as an autosomal dominant condition.
    C. the osmotic fragility test in HS produces a curve shifted to the left compared with normal cells.
    D. in HS the direct Coombs' test (antiglobulin) is positive.
    E. splenectomy is indicated in all cases.

46. **In childhood offensive loose stools may be caused by:**
    A. increased secretions of pancreatic enzymes.
    B. Bodian-Schwachmann syndrome.
    C. biliary atresia.
    D. cystic fibrosis.
    E. abetalipoproteinaemia.

47. **The following statements regarding galactosaemia are true:**
    A. can be diagnosed antenatally.
    B. has an incidence of 1 in 10 000 births.
    C. gives a positive result to a clinistix test of the urine.
    D. affected infants may be breastfed.
    E. treated infants will have IQs less than 100.

45. AB

In HS the osmotic fragility test curve is shifted to the right and the Coombs' test is negative. The presence of spherocytes and a positive Coombs' indicates an autoimmune haemolysis. Splenectomy is not always indicated and once performed necessitates prophylaxis against pneumococcal infections. Pigmentary gallstones are common in HS.

46. BCDE

A decrease or absence of pancreatic enzyme secretion may cause loose, offensive stools. Chest infections or respiratory signs are suggestive of cystic fibrosis. Bodian-Schwachmann syndrome presents with failure to thrive in the absence of respiratory symptoms, persistent neutropenia, thrombocytopenia, raised fetal haemoglobin and minor liver enzyme abnormalities. Growth retardation, skeletal dysostoses and bone marrow hypoplasia may also be present. Abetalipoproteinaemia results from a defective production of apoprotein B by the intestinal cells leading to defective synthesis of low-density lipoproteins, very low-density lipoproteins and chylomicrons (CLM). Absence of CLM results in fat malabsorption, deficiency of fat-soluble vitamins and steatorrhoea. Very low cholesterol (< 1.3 mmol/l), low triglyceride and acanthocytes on the blood film are found.

47. A

The enzyme deficiency (galactose-1-phosphate uridyl transferase) can be detected from chorionic villus sampling or from amniocentesis. The incidence is 1 in 50 000. Clintest tablets detect reducing substances in the urine. Clinistix are specific to detecting glucose. Treated individuals tend to have an IQ on average 10 points below that expected from the parents' average IQ.

48. **The following are examples of X-linked recessive disorders:**
    A. Hurler's syndrome.
    B. glucose-6-phosphate dehydrogenase (G6PD) deficiency.
    C. Becker muscular dystrophy.
    D. vitamin D resistant rickets.
    E. haemophilia B (Christmas disease).

49. **The following statements regarding cyanotic congenital heart disease are correct:**
    A. the most common aetiology is tetralogy of Fallot.
    B. a chest X-ray showing normal-sized heart, decreased pulmonary vascular markings and a boot-shaped heart is suggestive of transposition of the arteries.
    C. children with tetralogy of Fallot characteristically develop hypoxic spells between 6 and 12 months.
    D. when complete transposition of the arteries is present, often heart murmur is not detectable.
    E. cyanotic congenital heart disease often presents with acidosis, tachypnoea and poor feeding in the neonatal period.

50. **The umbilical artery:**
    A. is normally a single structure.
    B. is a branch of the internal iliac artery.
    C. passes through the liver.
    D. when catheterized may result in ischaemia of the buttocks.
    E. returns deoxygenated blood to the placenta *in utero*.

48. **BCDE**

    X-linked recessive disorders include:

    agammaglobulinaemia
    Becker muscular dystrophy
    chronic granulomatous disease
    Duchenne muscular dystrophy
    fragile X syndrome
    G6PD deficiency
    haemophilia A and B
    Hunter's disease (mucopolysaccharidosis type II)
    Lesch-Nyhan syndrome
    ornithine transcarbamolase deficiency
    vitamin D resistant rickets.

49. **ADE**

    The common causes of cyanotic congenital heart disease are tetralogy of Fallot and transposition of the great arteries. These two account for 10% and 6% of cyanotic congenital heart disease, respectively. Rarer causes include: total anomalous pulmonary venous drainage, tricuspid atresia, pulmonary atresia, Ebstein's anomaly, persistent truncus arteriosus, single ventricle and double outlet right ventricle. Each of these account for less than 1% of cyanotic congenital heart disease. Decreased pulmonary blood flow in tetralogy of Fallot results in oligaemic lung fields. A 'boot'-shaped heart can be seen on the X-ray in tetralogy of Fallot and is due to the concave shape of the main pulmonary artery segment. In complete transposition of the great arteries, no murmur is present unless an additional defect such as an atrial septal defect, ventricular septal defect, pulmonary stenosis or patent ductus arteriosus is present. Hypoxic spells occur at all ages.

50. **BDE**

    The umbilical artery is a bilateral structure and is a branch of the anterior division of the internal iliac artery. It ascends out of the pelvis along the anterior abdominal wall and joins the umbilicus. *In utero*, the umbilical arteries carry deoxygenated blood from the fetus to the placenta. The inferior gluteal artery is another branch of the anterior division of the internal iliac artery and it supplies blood to the skin over the buttocks. Umbilical artery cannulation may interfere with this supply and lead to ischaemia of this area.

51. **A 3-year-old girl presents for the first time with nephrotic syndrome. The following statements are correct:**
    A. prednisolone at 60 mg/m^2/day should be started.
    B. a renal biopsy should be carried out.
    C. one-third of children will have a single attack.
    D. C3 levels will probably be decreased.
    E. the most likely cause of nephrotic syndrome in this child is minimal change nephropathy.

52. **Normal development includes:**
    A. the presence of the Moro reflex at 3 months of age.
    B. being able to hop on one foot at the age of 3 years.
    C. the presence of a downward parachute by the age of 3 months.
    D. the presence of a forward parachute by the age of 7 months.
    E. hands being brought together in finger play by the age of 3 months.

53. **Pes cavus can be associated with:**
    A. spina bifida occulta.
    B. diastematomyelia.
    C. Friedreich's ataxia.
    D. Charcot-Marie-Tooth disease.
    E. Marfan syndrome.

51. ACE

Minimal change nephropathy, where there is fusion of the podocyte foot processes on electron microscopy, is the cause of nephrotic syndrome in about 90% of cases. Ninety-five per cent of children will respond to prednisolone at 60 $mg/m^2/day$ within 4 weeks. Response is said to have occurred when 3 days of protein-free urine are obtained. Renal biopsies are carried out if the presentation of nephrotic syndrome is atypical with gross haematuria or if the child is over 8 years old. The reason for the latter indication is that membranoproliferative and membranous glomerulonephritis become increasingly common over the age of 8 years. A further indication for a renal biopsy is in a child who is resistant to steroid therapy. Whilst one-third of children with minimal change nephropathy have only one attack, one-third will have infrequent relapses and one-third will have frequent relapses. Almost all remit by adulthood.

52. ADE

It is important to know about the primitive reflexes (Moro, rooting, grasp, asymmetric tonic neck reflex, etc.). All the primitive reflexes usually disappear by the age of 6 months as the child becomes able to sit and weight bear. A downward parachute appears at about 5 months of age and the forward parachute by the age of about 7 months. By the age of 3 years, a child can usually stand on one preferred foot momentarily when shown, and can hop on one foot by the age of 4 years.

53. ABCD

Spina bifida occulta is a benign insignificant finding in 20% of cases. There may be motor and sensory losses in the lower extremities and bladder and sphincter problems. This can lead to weaknesses in the small muscles in the feet resulting in pes cavus. Diastematomyelia can lead to tethering of the spinal cord resulting in progressive neurological deficit. Pes cavus is an early finding in Friedreich's ataxia. Charcot-Marie-Tooth disease or peroneal muscular atrophy is an autosomal dominant disorder that affects the nerves of the legs. Foot drop, peroneal myoatrophy and mild distal sensory impairment may be present. In Marfan syndrome the usual finding is pes planus.

54. In human skin:
  A. apocrine sweat glands produce secretions with a characteristic odour.
  B. apocrine glands are innervated by cholinergic sympathetic fibres.
  C. chondroitin sulphate is the main glycosaminoglycan (GAG) in the dermis.
  D. sebum consists of approximately equal amounts of free fatty acids, cholesterol and glycerides.
  E. a comedo is a blocked pilosebaceous gland.

55. Histamine has the following effects:
  A. vasoconstriction.
  B. bronchoconstriction.
  C. decreased gastric acid secretion.
  D. decreased intrinsic factor secretion.
  E. pruritis.

56. The following statements are correct:
  A. cow's milk has a higher protein content than breast milk.
  B. the calcium content of cow's milk is approximately three times that of an ordinary infant milk formula.
  C. cow's milk has less phosphate than breast milk.
  D. cow's milk and breast milk have approximately equal potassium contents.
  E. early introduction of cow's milk to an infant may result in hypocalcaemia.

57. In a 3-week-old baby with a serum bilirubin level of 275 μmol/l, the following findings support a diagnosis of breast milk jaundice:
  A. dark urine.
  B. conjugated bilirubin of 120 μmol/l.
  C. hepatomegaly.
  D. alkaline phosphatase of 400 IU/l.
  E. poor weight gain.

54. CE

Apocrine and eccrine glands are innervated by sympathetic fibres, the apocrine by adrenergic and the eccrine by cholinergic fibres. Apocrine secretions are odourless but the action of bacteria on the skin produces the foul smell of body odour. Chondroitin sulphate is the main GAG of the dermis. Sebum consists mainly of free fatty acids and glycerides; cholesterol is almost absent.

55. BE

Administration of histamine to the skin causes a wheal, flare and oedema (triple response). Histamine challenge may cause bronchoconstriction by stimulation of H1 receptors. Gastric acid, pepsinogen and intrinsic factor secretion is increased by stimulation of the H2 receptors.

56. ABE

The Composition of human milk, cow's milk and standard formula milk per 100 ml is shown in the table.

	Human breast milk	Unmodified cow's milk	Standard formula milk
Energy (kcal)	70.0	65.0	65.0
Carbohydrate (g)	7.0	4.7	7.2
Protein (g)	1.3	3.3	1.5
Fat (g)	4.2	3.8	3.6
Na (mmol)	0.65	2.17	0.78
K (mmol)	1.54	3.85	1.59
Ca (mmol)	0.88	3.0	1.2
PO_4 (mmol)	0.48	3.07	1.2
Fe (μmol)	1.36	0.9	12.0

57. All false

Breast milk jaundice can only be diagnosed after the exclusion of other serious causes of prolonged hyperbilirubinaemia. Breast milk contains steroids which may inhibit glucuronyl transferase. Babies with breast milk jaundice are well and have no evidence of obstructive jaundice (dark urine, pale stools). Conjugated bilirubin levels are less than 10% of the total bilirubin. The liver is not enlarged and serum liver enzyme concentrations are not raised.

58. **Congenital dislocation of the hip:**
    A. is more common in females.
    B. is more common after breech delivery.
    C. is more common in first-born infants.
    D. X-ray is useful to confirm the diagnosis.
    E. ultrasound is useful to confirm the diagnosis.

59. **The following are recognized causes of precocious puberty:**
    A. craniopharyngioma.
    B. Klinefelter syndrome.
    C. cimetidine therapy.
    D. pineal tumour.
    E. Turner's syndrome.

60. **The following statements regarding intussusception are correct:**
    A. adenovirus is a recognized cause.
    B. is more common in females.
    C. the ileocaecal site is the most common.
    D. never occurs in adults.
    E. passage of blood and mucus per rectum is an early sign.

58. **ABCE**

Congenital dislocation of the hip is approximately six times more common in females than males. Breech presentation occurs in 40% of cases and 60% are first-born infants. X-ray examination is not useful as the femoral head is uncalcified. Ultrasound examination may, however, be helpful in cases where clinical findings are in doubt.

59. **ACD**

Causes of precocious puberty:

True:	constitutional
	brain tumours (craniopharyngioma, pineal and hypothalamic tumours)
	hydrocephalus
	post-encephalitis
	neurofibromatosis
	tuberose sclerosis
	McCune-Albright syndrome
	hypothyroidism
	gonadotrophin secreting tumours (e.g. hepatoblastoma)
False:	congenital adrenal hyperplasia
	adrenal cortex tumours
	testicular tumours
	ovarian tumours.

60. **A**

Intussusception is more common in males and may be associated with infection with adenovirus and other viruses. Infants aged between 4 and 9 months are most commonly affected, but the condition may arise in older children and adults. The most common site is the lower ileum, forming the ileo-ileal variety. The passage of rectal blood and mucus is a late sign, heralding bowel ischaemia.

Paper 4

1. **Vitamin E deficiency:**
   A. is associated with retinopathy of prematurity.
   B. can cause cerebellar ataxia.
   C. is associated with abetalipoproteinaemia.
   D. may present with haemolytic anaemia.
   E. can be diagnosed by increased red blood cell haemolysis with hydrogen peroxide.

2. **The following statements about immunodeficiency are correct:**
   A. early onset (< 2 years) hypogammaglobulinaemia affects males and females equally.
   B. selective IgA deficiency is present in about 1 in 500 of the population.
   C. frequent infections with fungal and viral agents suggest a T-cell deficiency.
   D. chronic granulomatous disease (CGD) is usually an X-linked condition.
   E. in AIDS (acquired immunodeficiency syndrome) the CD4 to CD8 ratio increases.

3. **Radiological hallmarks of inflammatory bowel disease suggesting an underlying diagnosis of Crohn's disease are:**
   A. rose-thorn ulcers.
   B. fistulas.
   C. stricture.
   D. collar stud ulcers.
   E. shortened narrowed colon.

1. **ABCDE**
   Vitamin E acts as a biological reducing agent and prevents damage to cell membranes by high levels of oxygen. Premature infants absorb vitamin E poorly and this is thought to be one of the aetiological factors that lead to retinopathy of prematurity. Premature infants are also susceptible to haemolytic anaemia caused by vitamin E deficiency as another role of the vitamin is to stabilize red blood cell membranes. One of the diagnostic tests for vitamin E deficiency is that the red blood cells have an increased susceptibility to haemolysis by hydrogen peroxide. For this reason all premature infants should have vitamin E supplementation. Chronic vitamin E deficiency can lead to progressive areflexia, cerebellar ataxia and opthalmoplegia. Treatment is with tocopherol at a dose of 10 mg/kg/day. Owing to poor absorption this dose has to be increased to 100 mg/kg/day in abetalipoproteinaemia.

2. **BCD**
   Early hypogammaglobulinaemia is almost always the male sex-linked type (Bruton's). IgA deficiency is one of the most common immunodeficiencies. Abnormalities of cell-mediated immunity are less common than deficiencies of immunoglobulin. Frequent and severe viral and fungal infections or *Pneumocystis carinii* suggest a T-cell defect. A T-cell deficiency is found in Di George syndrome, Wiskott-Aldrich syndrome, ataxia telangiectasia and chronic mucocutaneous candidiasis. The CD4 to CD8 ratio decreases in AIDS.

3. **ABC**
   Collar stud ulcers occur in both ulcerative colitis and Crohn's disease and a shortened narrowed colon would suggest ulcerative colitis.

4. **In the hand:**
   A. damage to the radial nerve may produce wrist drop.
   B. the ulnar nerve supplies the opponens pollicis brevis muscle of the thumb.
   C. damage to the median nerve will result in wasting of the hypothenar eminence.
   D. the median nerve passes under the flexor retinaculum.
   E. the median nerve carries sensation from the medial half of the hand.

5. **In congenital diaphragmatic hernia (CDH):**
   A. hernias most commonly occur on the left.
   B. pulmonary hypoplasia is the major cause of death.
   C. persistent fetal circulation occurs uncommonly.
   D. associated congenital anomalies are common.
   E. most present between 12 and 24 hours of age.

4. **AD**

   Radial nerve damage secondary to a spiral groove fracture may produce wrist drop. The radial nerve supplies wrist and finger extensors. The ulnar nerve supplies sensation to the ulnar border of the hand and all the small muscles of the hand apart from the short flexors of the fingers, abductors and opponens of the thumb and lumbricals to the index and middle fingers. These are supplied by the median nerve. Sensation from the arm is carried by the nerve roots C5 to T1. The median nerve supplies sensation to the lateral half of the palm of the hand and the palmar aspect of the lateral three and one-half fingers, including the nail beds on the dorsum.

5. **AB**

   CDH is one of the most common neonatal surgical emergencies. The left side of the chest is more commonly affected than the right (4:1). Symptoms occur either from birth or shortly after the first feed. A more insidious presentation with increasing cough and tachypnoea has been described. Bilateral pulmonary hypoplasia, which is worse on the side of hernia, is the major cause of mortality. Antenatal diagnosis with aggressive resuscitation, ventilation and carefully timed surgery have improved survival. Persistent pulmonary hypertension and shunting of blood through the patent foramen ovale, ductus arteriosus and the lungs commonly occurs. It is usually an isolated defect.

6. **The following are recognized features of Turner's syndrome:**
   A. low birth weight.
   B. ovarian cysts.
   C. low plasma luteinizing hormone (LH) level.
   D. high plasma follicle-stimulating hormone (FSH) level.
   E. lymphoedema.

7. **The following are contraindications to breast feeding:**
   A. prematurity.
   B. maternal metronidazole therapy.
   C. maternal mastitis.
   D. cleft palate.
   E. galactosaemia.

8. **The following statements regarding messenger RNA (mRNA) are correct:**
   A. mRNA never contains introns.
   B. mRNA is translated into proteins in the nucleus.
   C. mRNA contains the bases cytosine and thymine.
   D. reverse transcriptase uses mRNA as a template to produce complementary DNA.
   E. mRNA is used in the Southern blotting technique.

6. ADE

The features of Turner's syndrome are:

low birth weight
short stature
short, webbed neck with low hair line and loose skin folds
typical facies (prominent ears, small jaw)
high arched palate
hypoplastic nails
oedema of hands and feet
shield-shaped chest
cubitus valgus
pigmented naevi
low IQ
hearing impairment
coarctation of the aorta
renal tract abnormalities
streak ovaries
high basal LH and FSH.

7. E

Mothers of preterm infants should be encouraged to breast feed their babies. If this is not possible expressed breast milk may be given. Maternal metronidazole therapy alters the taste of breast milk, but this is not a contraindication. Regular expression, either by continued feeding or pumping, should be recommended for maternal mastitis, along with analgesia and antibiotic treatment. Infants with a cleft palate can often breast feed. In some inborn errors of metabolism, breast milk must be excluded from the diet. These include galactosaemia, phenyl-ketonuria and alactasia.

8. D

The structure of mRNA is similar to DNA except that uracil replaces thymine as one of the bases. Both coding (exons) and non-coding regions of DNA are initially transcribed into mRNA. Splicing is required for mature mRNA to be produced only consisting of introns. Translation occurs in the cytoplasm. Southern blotting is a technique that uses denatured fragments of DNA in a gel to bind to DNA probes in order to detect the presence of particular genes or sequences of DNA. The enzyme reverse transcriptase can be used by viruses to insert viral mRNA into the host genome.

9. **The following are causes of bronchiectasis in childhood:**
   A. tuberculosis.
   B. whooping cough.
   C. measles.
   D. infectious mononucleosis.
   E. ciliary dyskinesia.

10. **Left axis deviation is seen on the ECG in the following conditions:**
    A. patent ductus arteriosus.
    B. Ebstein's anomaly.
    C. atrioventricular canal defects.
    D. large ventricular septal defect.
    E. tetralogy of Fallot.

11. **The following statements regarding hepatitis C are correct:**
    A. hepatitis C is a DNA virus.
    B. the major vector of transmission of hepatitis C is by the oro-faecal route.
    C. screening for hepatitis C is carried out when blood is donated in the UK.
    D. hepatitis C does not cause liver cirrhosis.
    E. interferon is used in the treatment of infected patients.

12. **The following are diagnostic criteria for Kawasaki's disease:**
    A. non-purulent conjunctivitis.
    B. polymorphic rash.
    C. cervical lymphadenopathy.
    D. polyarticular arthritis.
    E. fever for 3 or more days' duration.

13. **If Wood's light is shined on skin with the following conditions, affected areas fluoresce:**
    A. vitiligo.
    B. pityriasis rosea.
    C. tuberous sclerosis.
    D. hyperkeratotic eczema lesions.
    E. pityriasis versicolor.

9. **ABCE**
   Causes of bronchiectasis include:

   cystic fibrosis
   tuberculosis
   ciliary dyskinesia
   adenovirus infection
   whooping cough
   measles
   foreign body aspiration
   recurrent pulmonary infection.

10. **C**
    Left axis deviation is also seen in tricuspid atresia.

11. **CE**
    Hepatitis C is a single-stranded RNA virus. It is responsible for most non-A, non-B hepatitis infections post-blood transfusion. The incubation period of the virus is 6–12 weeks after a transfusion. There is a 50% chance of developing chronic aggressive hepatitis or cirrhosis following infection with hepatitis C. Prior to donating blood, serum is screened for the presence of anti-hepatitis C antibodies.

12. **ABC**
    Diagnostic criteria for Kawasaki's disease are:

    pyrexia for > 5 days
    non-purulent conjunctivitis
    mucous membrane changes
    desquamation of extremities
    polymorphous rash
    cervical lymphadenopathy
    coronary artery aneurysms.

13. **ACE**
    Wood's light produces fluorescence in skin infected by fungi, as in pityriasis versicolor, and in the hypopigmented patches of tuberous sclerosis and vitiligo. Pityriasis rosea is a common benign eruption that occurs in children and young adults. It is characterized by a herald patch followed by widespread ovoid lesions that may produce a 'Christmas tree' pattern on the back.

14. **The oxyhaemoglobin dissociation curve:**
    A. is shifted to the right by a decrease in pH.
    B. is shifted to the left by a decrease in temperature.
    C. is shifted to the right by a decrease in 2,3-diphosphoglyce-rate (2,3-DPG).
    D. is shifted to the right in haemoglobin F.
    E. is unaffected by exercise.

15. **The following are correct:**
    A. the median of a sample is the value that comes half way when data are ranked in order of magnitude.
    B. the smaller the standard deviation of a sample, the less the variation that is present in the sample.
    C. in a skewed distribution curve, 95% of the data lies within 1.96 × 2 standard deviations of the median.
    D. logarithmic transformation of skewed data may allow parametric analysis to be carried out on the data.
    E. interquantile ranges should be used to summarize the spread of skewed data.

16. **The following statements are correct:**
    A. the 1st pharyngeal arch gives rise to the mandible.
    B. the facial nerve develops in the 2nd pharyngeal arch.
    C. the 5th pharyngeal arch contains the vagus nerve.
    D. ectoderm from the 1st pharyngeal arch gives rise to the skin of the lower face and lips.
    E. the muscles of facial expression are derived from the 3rd pharyngeal arch.

14. **AB**

Oxygen is carried in the blood in two forms, dissolved (0.3 ml O_2/100 ml at a Po_2 of 100 mmHg) and in combination with haemoglobin (each gram of haemoglobin can combine with 1.39 ml O_2). For a haemoglobin of 15 g/100 ml the O_2 capacity is about 20.8 ml O_2/100 ml blood. Oxygen forms an easily reversible combination with haemoglobin to give oxyhaemoglobin. There is a rapid increase in the amount of O_2 carried by haemoglobin up to a Po_2 of about 50 mmHg after which the oxygen dissociation curve becomes flatter. The position of this curve is shifted by pH, Pco_2, and temperature, and a shift to the right results in unloading of O_2 to the peripheral tissue. In exercise muscle becomes acid, hypercapnoic and hot. All of these conditions help unload O_2. Under conditions of chronic hypoxia such as at high altitude or with any form of chronic lung disease, the red cell 2,3-DPG is increased, which shifts the curve to the right and aids unloading of oxygen. HbF shifts the curve to the left and HbS to the right.

Shift to right	Shift to left
Fall in pH	Rise in pH
Rise in Pco_2	Fall in Pco_2
Rise in temperature	Fall in temperature
Rise in 2,3-DPG	Fall in 2,3-DPG.

15. **ABDE**

When data have a skewed distribution curve it is not appropriate to use the mean and standard deviation to describe the data. The median and interquantile ranges should be used for this purpose. Logarithmic transformation may transform skewed data in order to create a symmetrical distribution curve so that parametric analysis may be performed.

16. **ABD**

There are six pharyngeal arches. The 5th arch disappears early. Each arch has its own nerve supply: arch 1, mandibular division of trigeminal nerve; 2, facial nerve; 3, glossopharyngeal nerve; 4, superior laryngeal branch of vagus; 6, recurrent laryngeal branch of vagus. The muscles of facial expression are derived from the 2nd arch.

17. **The following are features of acute intermittent porphyria:**
    A. positive Hoesch test.
    B. photosensitivity.
    C. autosomal recessive inheritance.
    D. diagnosed by the presence of gamma aminolaevulinic acid and porphobilinogen in the urine.
    E. a lack of symptoms until after puberty.

18. **A 5-year-old boy presents with signs of puberty. His testicular volume is 6 ml. The following conditions could account for this presentation:**
    A. hydrocephalus.
    B. 21-hydroxylase deficiency.
    C. neurofibromatosis.
    D. hepatoblastoma.
    E. McCune-Albright syndrome.

19. **A Meckel's diverticulum:**
    A. most frequently presents with haematemesis in children over 2 years.
    B. is situated on the anti-mesenteric surface of the gut.
    C. is a vestigial remnant of the vitello-intestinal duct.
    D. may contain ectopic gastric, pancreatic or colonic mucosa at the base.
    E. may form the apex of an ileo-ileal intussusception.

20. **The following statements are correct:**
    A. insulin is derived from C-peptide.
    B. glucagon stimulates insulin release.
    C. C-peptide levels are increased in endogenous hyperinsulinaemia.
    D. insulin decreases absorption of glucose from the gut.
    E. catecholamines antagonize the actions of insulin.

17. **AD**

The porphyrias are a group of illnesses caused by a deficiency of one of the seven enzymes involved in haem biosynthesis. Acute intermittent porphyria is caused by porphobilinogen deaminase deficiency. It is diagnosed by the presence of gamma aminolaevulinic acid and porphobilinogen in the urine. The Hoesch test detects porphobilinogen in the urine by turning a cherry-red colour. Symptoms of the illness may start prior to puberty.

18. **ACD**

The boy has 'true' precocious puberty as he has an increased testicular volume (normal <2ml) as well as signs of puberty. Hydrocephalus and neurofibromatosis can cause precocious puberty as a result of premature activation of the hypothalamic-pituitary-gonadal axis. Human chorionic gonadotrophin can be produced by hepatoblastoma causing premature maturation of the testis. In 21-hydroxylase deficiency there are signs of puberty but testicular volume is appropriate for age. McCune-Albright syndrome is the association of endocrine dysfunction with polyostotic fibrous dysplasia and abnormal pigmentation. Although it is seen in boys it does not cause premature puberty.

19. **BCE**

Meckel's diverticulum occurs in 2–3% of the population and is usually about 60 cm proximal to the ileocaecal junction on the anti-mesenteric surface of the gut. This remnant of the vitello-intestinal duct most frequently presents with painless rectal bleeding with a peak incidence of symptoms in the first 2 years of life. The mucosal lining is the same as the adjacent ileum but more than 35% have ectopic gastric, pancreatic or colonic mucosa at the tip. Presentation is either with painless rectal bleeding or abdominal pain resulting from diverticulitis or an intussusception.

20. **BCE**

Insulin is derived from proinsulin, which is cleaved to form insulin and C-peptide. C-peptide can be measured to distinguish between endogenous hyperinsulinaemia and exogenously administered insulin. Insulin inhibits glucagon release, whereas glucagon stimulates insulin release. Insulin has no effect on the absorption of glucose from the gut. Catecholamines inhibit the action of insulin.

21. A term infant has a serum bilirubin of 331 mmol/l (unconjugated 310 mmol/l) and a haemoglobin of 8.8 g/dl at 10 days of age. The baby's blood group is A Rhesus negative and the mother's blood group is O Rhesus positive. The direct Coombs test is negative. Phototherapy is started and group O Rhesus negative donor red blood cells are transfused. The bilirubin is found to be 351 mmol/l 6 hours later. The following are diagnostic possibilities:
    A. physiological jaundice.
    B. Rhesus incompatibility.
    C. ABO incompatibility.
    D. Crigler-Najjar syndrome.
    E. transfusion mismatch.

22. The following infections are caused by gram-positive organisms:
    A. whooping cough.
    B. typhoid.
    C. diphtheria.
    D. ophthalmia neonatorum.
    E. tetanus.

23. A boy of 2 years cannot walk yet. Duchenne muscular dystrophy is unlikely if:
    A. there is no family history of Duchenne muscular dystrophy.
    B. the serum creatine phosphokinase (CPK) is 236 IU/l.
    C. facial muscle weakness is present.
    D. a muscle biopsy is normal.
    E. hyperreflexia is present.

21. AC

The infant has hyperbilirubinaemia and anaemia, suggesting haemolysis. The mother is Rhesus positive and so Rhesus isoimmunization is not possible. As she is blood group O she has anti-A and anti-B antibodies (IgG) which can cross the placenta and cause haemolysis of the infant's red blood cells. Crigler-Najjar syndrome type I is an autosomal recessive condition leading to absence of uridyl diphosphoglucuronyl transferase (UDPGT). Severe unconjugated hyperbilirubinaemia occurs in the neonatal period. Although haemolysis does not occur as part of this syndrome, this unlikely diagnosis cannot be excluded using the information given in the question. Physiological jaundice presents after the first 24 hours of life, reaches a peak between the 3rd and 5th day at a maximum level of 200–250 μmol/l and disappears by the 10th to 14th day. Group O blood is considered the universal donor.

22. CE

Causative organisms are as follows:

whooping cough	– *Bordetella pertussis*
typhoid	– *Salmonella typhi*
diphtheria	– *Corynebacterium diphtheriae*
ophthalmia neonatorum	– *Neisseria gonorrhoeae*
tetanus	– *Clostridium tetani*

Refer to table in Question 43, Paper 2.

23. BCDE

Approximately one-third of cases of Duchenne muscular dystrophy are new mutations with no past family history of the disease. The legs usually have moderate proximal weakness at the time of presentation, but upper limb and facial musculature may appear relatively normal for several more years. The serum CPK is grossly elevated (>1000 IU/l) and muscle biopsy confirms the diagnosis.

24. **The following statements regarding the diagnosis and management of an ostium secundum atrial septal defect (ASD) are correct:**
    A. fixed splitting of the second heart sound suggests the presence of an ASD.
    B. right bundle branch block (RBBB) with an rSR pattern in lead V1 can be seen on the ECG of a child with an ASD.
    C. the child can expect mild symptoms.
    D. spontaneous closure of an ASD may occur in up to 40% of cases in the first 5 years of life.
    E. atrial arrhythmias can occur in adult life if the defect is untreated.

25. **These statements relating to normal development are correct:**
    A. a 2-year-old can turn pages one at a time.
    B. at 15 months a child can build a tower of six cubes.
    C. a squint at 6 months is definitely abnormal.
    D. a 1 year old can retrieve a toy hidden before his or her eyes under a cup or cushion.
    E. at 5 years a child can copy a square but not a triangle.

26. **The following are recognized signs of child sexual abuse:**
    A. reflex anal dilatation.
    B. enuresis in a child who has previously been continent at night.
    C. a sudden deterioration in school performance.
    D. inappropriate sexual knowledge.
    E. laboratory evidence of *Chlamydia trachomatis* in a vaginal swab.

27. **In vascular endothelium:**
    A. nitric oxide (NO) is produced from citrulline by the action of enzyme nitric oxide synthatase (NOS).
    B. endothelial derived relaxing factor (EDRF) is the molecule NO.
    C. NO produces vasorelaxation by increasing cGMP production.
    D. released endogenous NO has a half-life of about 20 seconds.
    E. tachyphylaxis in the pulmonary circulation commonly occurs when NO is used as an inhaled therapy.

24. ABDE

The secundum ASD is due to a defect in the atrial septum, the site of the fossa ovalis. A defect near the entrance of the superior rena cava or inferior vena cava to the right atrium is a sinus venous type. An ECG shows right axis deviation (+90 to +180) and mild right ventricular hypertrophy or RBBB with an rSR pattern in V1. In the third and fourth decades of life pulmonary hypertension, congestive heart failure and atrial arrhythmias may occur.

25. ACDE

A child at 15 months, when given a book, will look at the pictures and pat pages. At 18 months he/she will look at the pictures and turn several pages. A child of 2 years should be able to turn pages one at a time. A child at 15 months can usually build a 2-cube tower; at 18 months, a 3-cube tower; at 2 years, a 6-cube tower; at 2½ years, a 7-cube tower and by 3 years, a 9-cube tower. A child at 15 months can usually grasp a crayon and imitate to-and-fro scribble; at 18 months can spontaneously make to-and-fro scribble with either hand; at 2 years can make circular scribble; at 2½ years can draw vertical and horizontal lines, circles + T and V shapes; at 3 years can copy circles; at 4 years can copy a cross; at 5 years can copy a square and at 5½ years can copy a triangle. By 6 months full conjugate eye movement is present and the slightest squint is abnormal.

26. BCDE

Reflex anal dilatation is not exclusively found in child sex abuse. It is also commonly seen in children with constipation and is now rarely used in the diagnosis of child sex abuse.

27. BC

Arginine under the action of NOS gives rise to NO and citrulline. EDRF has been shown to be the molecule NO, which has a free radical structure with an extra electron. For this reason it is short lived with a half-life of about 6–7 seconds. Tachyphylaxis has rarely been reported.

28. **The following drugs can cause bronchospasm:**
    A. captopril.
    B. atenolol.
    C. salmeterol.
    D. ibuprofen.
    E. paracetamol.

29. **A child has had a splenectomy following traumatic splenic rupture in a road traffic accident. The following may be present on the blood film six months later:**
    A. thrombocytosis.
    B. eliptocytosis.
    C. Howell-Jolly bodies.
    D. macrocytosis.
    E. fragmented cells.

30. **In childhood pulmonary tuberculosis:**
    A. sputum cultures are positive for tubercle bacilli in most cases.
    B. a reduced or absent Mantoux test occurs in HIV infection.
    C. steroid treatment does not affect the Mantoux test.
    D. chest X-ray may be normal.
    E. primary infection is more common in the upper lobes in young children.

31. **The following statements are true:**
    A. the renal arteries branch from the aorta at the level of the 4th and 5th lumbar vertebrae.
    B. the superior mesenteric artery branches from the aorta at the level of the 1st and 2nd lumbar vertebrae.
    C. an umbilical artery catheter (UAC) tip should ideally be placed in the left atrium.
    D. the umbilical vein is a single structure.
    E. a UAC appears more anterior than an umbilical venous catheter on a lateral abdominal X-ray.

28. CD

One side-effect of captopril is a persistent cough which is not due to bronchoconstriction. Atenolol is a cardioselective beta-blocker. Salmeterol is a beta-2 agonist and has a significant incidence of paradoxical bronchospasm. Non-steroidal anti-inflammatory agents should be avoided in children with asthma.

29. AC

The spleen removes intracytoplasmic inclusions such as Howell-Jolly bodies, Heinz bodies and siderotic granules. All of these are increased after splenectomy. Senescent cells are removed by the spleen and when it is absent the red cells are flatter and thinner than normal, target cells and spherocytes are increased and osmotic fragility is decreased. There are also depressed levels of IgM, properidin and tuftsin (which promotes phagocytosis).

30. BD

Primary pulmonary tuberculosis is more common in the lower lobes in younger children but more likely to be in the upper lobes in older children. The chest X-ray may be normal, show hilar lymphadenopathy, consolidation or miliary disease. Steroid therapy or HIV infection may lead to a decreased or absent reaction to tuberculin in the Mantoux test. Sputum cultures are positive in a minority of paediatric cases of tuberculosis.

31. BD

It is important to know the branches of the aorta when inserting UACs:

coeliac axis	– level of T12–L1
superior mesenteric artery	– level of L1–L2
renal arteries	– level of L1–L2
inferior mesenteric artery	– level of L2–L3

UACs can either be sited so that the tip lies in the aorta at the level of T6–T10 (high position) or L4 (low position). A lateral chest and abdominal X-ray shows the UAC in the aorta, and therefore posterior to an umbilical venous catheter.

32. **Medical indications for circumcision in children include:**
   A. hypospadias.
   B. recurrent urinary tract infections.
   C. recurrent ballanitis.
   D. ambiguous genitalia.
   E. cryptorchidism.

33. **Macrocephaly can be present in the following conditions:**
   A. Tay-Sachs' disease.
   B. thalassaemia major.
   C. Sotos syndrome.
   D. Rett syndrome.
   E. Hurler syndrome.

34. **The following are recognized causes of acute interstitial nephritis in children:**
   A. phenytoin.
   B. cytomegalovirus (CMV).
   C. sarcoidosis.
   D. transplant rejection.
   E. captopril.

32. BC
Circumcision is contraindicated in hypospadiasis since the tissue of the foreskin may be required for urethral reconstruction. Circumcision should be considered in the setting of recurrent urinary tract infections. Recurrent ballanitis is a clear indication for circumcision.

33. ABCE
It is important to measure parental head circumferences before a diagnosis of macrocephaly can be made. The average head circumference increases by 1 cm/month for the first year and then by about 1 cm/year. Children with Sotos syndrome or cerebral gigantism have accelerated growth for the first 4–5 years and then a normal rate of growth. A degree of mental retardation is present in most children with the condition as well as an increased predisposition to malignancies. Microcephaly is typically present in children with Rett syndrome.

34. ABCD
Interstitial nephritis is defined as inflammation between glomeruli in areas surrounding the tubules. There are many causes, which can be divided into acute or chronic:

Acute: **Drugs** – penicillins, sulphonamides, cotrimoxazole, rifampicin, phenytoin, thiazides, frusemide, allopurinol, cimetidine
Infections – streptococcal, pyelonephritis, toxoplasmosis, diphtheria, brucellosis, leptospirosis, infectious mononucleosis, CMV
Diseases – sarcoidosis, glomerulonephritis, transplant rejection
Chronic: **Drugs** – analgesics, lithium
Infections – pyelonephritis
Diseases – vesico-ureteric reflux, nephrocalcinosis, prolonged hypokalaemia, oxalate nephropathy, heavy metals, radiation, obstructive uropathy, medullary cystic disease.

35. **The following statements are correct:**
    A. prothrombin time is used to assess the extrinsic pathway.
    B. prothrombin time is increased in haemophilia A.
    C. prolonged bleeding time is a feature of von Willebrand's disease.
    D. von Willebrand's disease has X-linked inheritance.
    E. haemarthrosis is a common feature of Henoch-Schonlein purpura.

36. **Ventricular septal defects (VSDs):**
    A. affect the membranous septum most commonly.
    B. only cause the Eisenmenger syndrome in adulthood.
    C. are usually associated with a normal ECG.
    D. rarely cause infective endocarditis.
    E. are not associated with a diastolic murmur.

37. **In a new test to diagnose sepsis in newborn infants, 100 infants are tested and the test results compared with subsequent blood culture results. Nineteen out of 50 infants with a positive test also had a positive blood culture. One infant out of 50 with a negative test result had a positive blood culture. The following statements are true:**
    A. the sensitivity of the test is 95%.
    B. the specificity of the test is 95%.
    C. the positive predictive value is the same as the sensitivity.
    D. the negative predictive value is 98%.
    E. the prevalence of sepsis in infants tested is 20%.

38. **The following statements regarding secretory IgA (sIgA) are correct:**
    A. sIgA has a molecular weight of 140 kDa.
    B. sIgA exists as a dimeric molecule.
    C. sIgA is unable to fix complement.
    D. sIgA contains a J chain.
    E. sIgA makes up 10% of the circulating immunoglobulins present in the serum.

35. AC

Prothrombin time is an assessment of the extrinsic and common pathway. It is normal in haemophilia A and B and also von Willebrand's disease. The activated partial thromboplastic time (APTT) and bleeding time are increased in von Willebrand's disease, which is inherited as an autosomal dominant trait with variable expression. Periarticular swelling may occur with Henoch-Schonlein purpura but haemarthrosis is not usually a feature of the illness.

36. ACD

Eisenmenger syndrome may occur in childhood if the defect is large. A diastolic flow murmur may occur with a large VSD because of increased flow across the mitral valve. Infective endocarditis is a complication in approximately 1% of cases. The ECG is usually normal, but may show biventricular hypertrophy.

37. ADE

See Question 44, Paper 3.

38. BD

IgA is present in the monomeric form in the serum. It makes up 10% of the circulating immunoglobulins and has a molecular weight of 140 kDa. Secretory IgA exists as a dimer with a J or joining chain connecting the two molecules together. The combined molecular weight of this molecule is 400 kDa. Secretory IgA is not present in the serum but is found in breast milk and is secreted by mucous surfaces such as the lung. Unlike IgA found in the serum, secretory IgA is able to fix complement. Secretory IgA also contains a secretory piece which allows the immunoglobulin to resist proteolysis.

39. The following conditions show a predisposition to developing hepatocellular carcinoma:
A. tyrosinaemia.
B. galactosaemia.
C. alpha-1 antitrypsin deficiency.
D. hepatitis A.
E. beta-thalaessaemia.

40. In a child who has accidentally ingested a poison, vomiting should not be induced in the following conditions:
A. >4 hours have elapsed since the ingestion.
B. ingestion of bleach.
C. ingestion of paraffin.
D. no gag reflex present in the child.
E. ingestion of aspirin.

41. The *Haemophilus influenzae* type B vaccine (Hib) vaccine:
A. is a live attenuated vaccine.
B. is recommended for children aged between 2 months and 4 years.
C. needs to be given as three doses in all children.
D. is very effective.
E. is contraindicated if there is a history of egg allergy in the family.

39. ABCE

Hepatocellular carcinoma is found frequently in conditions where liver cirrhosis is an important feature. Serum alpha-fetoprotein is raised in up to 80% of cases. Prognosis for children with this condition is poor.

40. BCD

There are several contraindications to inducing emesis after ingestion of a poison. (1) >4 hours since the ingestion unless the substance slows down gastric emptying, e.g. aspirin or tricyclic antidepressants. (2) If the substance is corrosive vomiting will cause further damage to the gastric mucosa. (3) If the substance is volatile, e.g. paraffin, turpentine or petrol, there is a risk of inhalation. (4) If the child is unconscious and has no gag reflex.

41. BD

Hib is a capsular conjugated polysaccharide vaccine. It is generally given in a course of three doses at monthly intervals at 2, 3 and 4 months with the other routine vaccinations. Over 13 months and up to 4 years a single dose is effective. As the risk of invasive *Haemophilus* falls rapidly after 4 years, it is only given after this age to those children considered to be at increased risk of invasive *Haemophilus* disease (sickle cell disease, antineoplastic therapy, an absent spleen). It is known to be highly effective but vaccination failures have been reported. Hypersensitivity to egg contraindicates influenza vaccines. Evidence of previous anaphylactic reaction contraindicates the use of the MMR and yellow fever vaccines.

42. **Failure to thrive may be caused by:**
    A. sensitivity to the gliadin fraction of gluten in the colon.
    B. psychological problems.
    C. introduction of cow's milk into the diet.
    D. a congenital deficiency of lactase.
    E. asthma.

43. **The following statements regarding Klinefelter syndrome are correct:**
    A. 99% of males with the condition have impaired spermatogenesis.
    B. gynaecomastia is frequently present.
    C. decreased luteinizing hormone (LH)/follicle-stimulating hormone (FSH) levels are present.
    D. mental handicap can be found in most cases.
    E. a Barr body can be present in the nuclei of cells in boys with the syndrome.

44. **The following statements are true:**
    A. secretion of parathyroid hormone (PTH) is stimulated by increased ionized calcium levels in extracellular fluid.
    B. vitamin D increases calcium and phosphate mobilization from bone.
    C. vitamin D increases calcium and phosphate absorption from the intestine.
    D. PTH increases reabsorption of phosphate from the proximal renal tubule.
    E. calcitonin is secreted by thyroid C-cells.

42. **BCD**

Coeliac disease is caused by a sensitivity to the gliadin fraction of gluten in the duodenum and jejunum. It is well established that emotional deprivation can cause growth failure. Persistent diarrhoea and growth failure may occur following the introduction of cow's milk into the diet. A soya based or hydrolysed casein milk (e.g. pregestimil) may be used in this situation. It must be remembered that about 40% of infants that are intolerant to cow's milk protein are also intolerant to the soya protein. Chronic diarrhoea can be due to either a post-gastroenteritis lactase deficiency or a primary lactase deficiency. The latter is more likely to be associated with abnormal growth and malabsorption. In either case the stools will be positive for reducing substances (Clinitest positive) and a low-lactose milk (e.g. pregestimil, galactomin, wysoy, nutramigen) should be used in treatment.

43. **ABE**

Most children with Klinefelter syndrome have the karyotype 47, XXY. Microrchidism, azospermia and sterility are almost always present. Elevated levels of LH and FSH are present owing to the low levels of testosterone. The diagnosis is rarely made before puberty although behavioural problems may be apparent long before defects in sexual development are noted. IQ is normal in most children with the syndrome. In individuals with 48, XXXY or 49, XXXXY, there may be two or three Barr bodies present.

44. **BCE**

PTH is stimulated by low levels of ionized calcium in extracellular fluid. It leads to increased mobilization of calcium and phosphate from bone and increases calcium from the distal renal tubule. PTH also inhibits reabsorption of phosphate from the proximal renal tubule. The biologically active form of vitamin D (1,25-hydroxycholecalciferol) increases mobilization of calcium and phosphate from bone and increases gut absorption of calcium and phosphate. Calcitonin is secreted by thyroid C-cells and inhibits bone resorption in response to increased calcium.

45. The following drugs are appropriately linked to substances that reverse their action:
  A. morphine — naloxone.
  B. warfarin — protamine.
  C. pancuronium — neostigmine.
  D. propanolol — isoprenaline.
  E. ipratropium bromide — atropine.

46. The following statements regarding the development of the respiratory system in the fetus are correct:
  A. the lung bud appears between the weeks 3 and 5 as an endodermal outgrowth of the foregut.
  B. in the pseudoglandular period airways grow by dichotomous divisions.
  C. lung cartilage appears from 16 weeks.
  D. the respiratory bronchioles develop from 24 weeks.
  E. the acinus consists of the last three airway generations.

47. Complications of cystic fibrosis include:
  A. biliary cirrhosis.
  B. nasal polyps.
  C. constipation.
  D. diabetes mellitus.
  E. rectal prolapse.

48. The following statements regarding sudden infant death syndrome (SIDS) are correct:
  A. the incidence is equal for infants born prematurely and at term.
  B. it occurs more commonly in lower socio-economic groups.
  C. if parents smoke, there is a two-fold increased risk of a baby dying as a result of SIDS.
  D. SIDS does not occur after 6 months of age.
  E. siblings of children who suffered SIDS have a five-fold increased chance of dying from SIDS.

45. **ACD**

    Naloxone is a narcotic antagonist that competes for central nervous system narcotic receptor sites. Protamine combines with heparin to form a complex without anticoagulant activity. Neostigmine inhibits acetylcholinesterase at the neuromuscular junction, thereby reversing the action of non-depolarizing muscle relaxants such as pancuronium, which competitively block cholinergic receptors. Propanolol is a non-selective beta-blocker and isoprenaline is a beta agonist. Ipratropium bromide (Atrovent) is an atropine derivative.

46. **ABE**

    The lung bud appears in the embryonic period between 3 and 5 weeks as an outgrowth of the foregut. During the pseudogland-ular period, 6–16 weeks, all the conducting airways from trachea to terminal bronchioles develop, i.e. the preacinus. Lung cartilage appears with the lymphatics at 10 weeks, and cilia at 10–13 weeks. The respiratory bronchioles and alveoli ducts develop during the canalicular period, 17–24 weeks. The acinus consists of the respiratory bronchioli, alveolar ducts and alveolar sacs.

47. **ABCDE**

    Symptomatic cirrhosis occurs in 2–3% of patients with cystic fibrosis; 25% have changes at post-mortem in the liver. Nasal polyps are common (15–20%). Constipation can be due to: excessive pancreatic supplements, meconium ileus equivalent, intestinal stricture secondary to pancreatic supplements or intussusception. Diabetes mellitus may occur at any age and is not related to the disease severity. It is often mild and may not need insulin therapy. Rectal prolapse occurs most frequently in infants and is related to steatorrhoea, malnutrition and repetitive cough.

48. **BCE**

    If babies are left to sleep in the prone position there is an increased risk of SIDS. There is an increased incidence of SIDS in premature infants, low-birth-weight infants and siblings of SIDS victims. It is more common in lower socio-economic groups. Parental smoking (maternal > paternal) is also a risk factor. Peak incidence is around 3–4 months and most cases occur before 6 months of age although it has been reported up to 1 year.

49. **The following conditions show the characteristics of genetic anticipation:**
    A. Huntington's chorea.
    B. von Willebrand's disease.
    C. cystic fibrosis.
    D. fragile X syndrome.
    E. dystrophia myotonica.

50. **The following ocular associations are correct:**
    A. retinal detachment   – Ehlers-Danlos syndrome.
    B. lens dislocation   – Marfan's syndrome.
    C. retinitis pigmentosa   – abetalipoproteinaemia.
    D. Kayser-Fleischer (KF) ring   – Down's syndrome.
    E. buphthalmos   – Lowe's syndrome.

51. **The following are characteristic of rickets of prematurity:**
    A. commoner in formula-fed infants.
    B. abnormal vitamin D metabolism.
    C. inadequate phosphate intake.
    D. alkaline phosphatase level greater than 500 IU/l.
    E. large anterior fontanelle.

49. ADE

In Huntington's chorea, fragile X syndrome and dystrophia myotonica, symptoms of the disease become increasingly severe as the genes carrying the condition are passed on from one generation to the next. This is called genetic anticipation. In cases of dystrophia myotonica and fragile X syndrome the manifestations of the disease are worse if the gene is passed on by the maternal carrier. The mechanism by which this happens has been shown to be due to repeated segments of DNA. The number of these repeated segments increases as the gene is passed on until a critical number of repeats are present and the condition is expressed.

50. ABCE

Ocular defect	Cause/condition
Corneal clouding/opacity	Hypoparathyroidism, Fabry's disease, cystinosis, Wilson's disease (KF ring), mucopolysaccharidosis
Lens dislocation	Homocystinuria (down), Marfan's disease (upward)
Cataract	galactosaemia, fructosaemia, phenylketonuria, Lowe's syndrome
Peripheral retinal degeneration (retinitis pigmentosa)	Tay-Sachs' disease, abetalipoproteinaemia, San Fillipo syndrome, Refsum's disease, hyperlipidaemia type I
Central retinal degeneration	Gangliosidosis, Tay-Sachs' disease, Gaucher's disease, Niemann-Pick disease
Retinal detachment	Marfan's syndrome, Ehlers-Danlos syndrome, buphthalmos.

51. CDE

Breast milk contains inadequate amounts of phosphate (and calcium) and this must either be supplemented or vitamin D supplements given, in order to prevent osteopenia (rickets) in preterm infants. Clinical features may include prolonged ventilator dependency, pain with handling, pathological fractures, widened ends of long bones, rachitic rosary and soft skull bones (craniotabes) with widening of sutures and enlargement of fontanelles.

52. Congenital adrenal hyperplasia (CAH):
   A. has presenting features that result from excessive adreno-corticotrophic hormone (ACTH) secretion.
   B. has an incidence of about 1 in 10 000.
   C. is most commonly due to 17-hydroxylase (17-OH) deficiency.
   D. may present with hyponatraemia, hypochloridaemia and hypokalaemia.
   E. can be diagnosed by increased plasma 17-OH progesterone levels.

53. The following statements are correct:
   A. the potency of a drug is the capacity of the drug to produce an effect and refers to the maximum such effect.
   B. the therapeutic index of a drug is a measure of the safety of a drug.
   C. in first-order pharmacokinetics, the rate of drug distribution is proportional to the concentration of the drug.
   D. for the half-life of a drug to be constant, first-order pharmacokinetics need to be present.
   E. phase I metabolism involves the conjugation of a drug with a molecule in order to ensure elimination of the drug.

52. **AE**

    CAH is a variable clinical syndrome caused by an ACTH-driven adrenocortical hypersecretion secondary to an enzyme deficiency. Decreased cortisol production results in a loss of negative feedback to the hypothalamic-pituitary axis and thus increased ACTH secretion. Incidence of the condition is about 1 in 5000 births. 21-hydroxylase deficiency is the common variant of CAH accounting for up to 95% of cases. A variable proportion (approximately 50%) of the 21-hydroxylase deficient type have salt-losing crises. The biochemical features of a salt-losing crisis are: metabolic acidosis, hyponatraemia, hypochloridaemia, hyperkalaemia, hypoglycaemia and hyperuraemia. Treatment includes glucocorticoid and mineralocorticoid replacement. Increased plasma 17-OH progesterone is a feature of 21-hydroxylase deficiency along with increased urine free cortisol, increased urinary 17-oxosteroids and urinary pregnantriol.

53. **BCD**

    The potency of a drug is the amount of the drug in relation to its effect. The efficacy of a drug is the capacity of the drug to produce an effect and refers to the maximum such effect. The therapeutic index can be defined in animals as LD_{50}/ED_{50} (LD_{50}= lethal dose in 50% of animals; ED_{50}= effective dose in 50% of animals). In humans the dose of a drug that gives unwanted side-effects is substituted in place of the LD_{50}. Drugs undergo absorption, distribution, metabolism and excretion. In most cases the rates at which these processes occur are proportional to the concentration of the drug. This is called first-order pharmacokinetics. When the rate of elimination of a drug follows first-order pharmacokinetics the time taken for the concentration of the drug to fall to half its value, from any concentration, is constant. Phase I metabolism involves a change of a drug molecule by oxidation, reduction or hydrolysis. Phase II metabolism involves the conjugation of a drug with a water-soluble molecule. The conjugates can be glucuronic acid, sulphate, acetyl coenzyme A or glutathione. Excretion occurs either via the kidney or, if the molecular weight is greater than 300, in the bile.

54. **Absent ankle reflexes and extensor plantar reflexes are seen in the following conditions:**
   A. abetalipoproteinaemia.
   B. cord compression at L3/L4.
   C. metachromatic leukodystrophy.
   D. Friedreich's ataxia.
   E. vitamin B_{12} deficiency.

55. **A 6-year-old boy has a 2-week history of being generally unwell. He presents with abdominal pain, arthritis and a widespread rash over his legs and buttocks. A diagnosis of Henoch-Schonlein purpura (HSP) would be supported by the following findings:**
   A. a low platelet count.
   B. the rash distribution being centrifugal.
   C. a vasculitis affecting large muscular arteries being present.
   D. the rash being purpuric in nature.
   E. the presence of haematuria.

56. **The daily recommended intake in the first year of life includes:**
   A. vitamin C   –   30 mg.
   B. vitamin D   –   1000 IU.
   C. fluids   –   85 ml/kg .
   D. calories   –   110 kcal/kg.
   E. protein   –   2 g/kg.

54. ACDE

The clinical presentation of absent ankle reflexes and extensor plantar reflexes suggests a combination of upper and lower motor neuron signs. In abetalipoproteinaemia, metachromatic leukodystrophy, Friedreich's ataxia and vitamin B_{12} deficiency there are combinations of corticospinal tract dysfunction and peripheral neuropathy which result in the mixed upper and lower motor neuron signs. In spinal cord compression at L3/L4 there will be a loss of the knee jerk reflex. The ankle jerk reflex will be intact.

55. BE

HSP is the most common form of non-thrombocytopenic purpura, the rash having a centrifugal distribution on the limbs rather than the trunk. The rash in HSP is vasculitic. The vasculitis of HSP affects the small non-muscular arterioles, capillaries and venules. A vasculitis of the large muscular arteries suggests polyarteritis nodosa. Renal involvement occurs in 25–50% of HSP.

56. ADE

Vitamin requirements (per day) for infants are as follows:

vitamin A	–	1500 IU
thiamine	–	0.3–0.5 mg
riboflavin	–	0.4–0.6 mg
vitamin C	–	30–35 mg
vitamin D	–	400 IU (10 mg)
vitamin E	–	3–4 mg.

Daily fluid requirement for infants after the first week is 150 ml/kg for term infants and up to 200 ml/kg for preterm infants, until weaning, and then 100–120 ml/kg.
Energy requirement is 115 kcal/kg/day for the first 6 months and then 105 kcal/kg/day from 6–12 months.
Protein requirement for infants is 2–2.2 g/kg/day.

57. The following are recognized causes of recurrent abdominal pain in childhood:
   A. duodenal ulcer.
   B. splenic infarction.
   C. lead poisoning.
   D. acute intermittent porphyria.
   E. ovarian cyst.

58. Acute epiglottitis:
   A. is most commonly caused by *Haemophilus influenzae* type A.
   B. beta-haemolytic streptococcus is a recognized cause.
   C. often recurs.
   D. diagnosis is often aided by a lateral neck X-ray.
   E. treatment of choice is ampicillin.

57. ABCDE

Non-organic or 'functional' causes account for over 90% of children with recurrent abdominal pain. The diagnoses listed below are all uncommon:

> peptic ulceration
> coeliac disease
> inflammatory bowel disease
> food allergies
> intermittent subacute obstruction (malrotation, adhesions, etc.)
> recurrent urinary tract infection
> renal/bladder calculi
> gallstones
> cholecystitis
> chronic pancreatitis
> chronic hepatitis
> cystic fibrosis
> diabetes
> porphyrias
> lead poisoning.

58. B

Acute epiglottitis is most commonly caused by *Haemophilus influenzae* type B but may be caused by beta-haemolytic streptococcus, pneumococcus *or Staphylococcus aureus*. Unlike laryngotracheobronchitis ('croup'), acute epiglottitis rarely recurs. A lateral neck X-ray is not recommended as this may delay diagnosis and neck extension may precipitate acute obstruction of the upper airway. *Haemophilus influenzae* may be resistant to ampicillin and therefore the antibiotic treatment of choice is either chloramphenicol or a third-generation cephalosporin.

59. **Third generation cephalosporins:**
   A. are principally excreted by the kidney.
   B. are effective treatment for *Staphylococcus aureus* infections.
   C. are effective against beta-lactamase-producing *Huemophilus influenzae.*
   D. cause adverse reactions in over 30% of patients with known penicillin hypersensitivity.
   E. are the treatment of choice for Pseudomonas colonization of the lung in cystic fibrosis.

60. **The following conditions cause an increased anion gap:**
   A. diabetic ketoacidosis.
   B. proximal renal tubular acidosis.
   C. aspirin poisoning.
   D. lactic acidosis.
   E. acute renal failure.

59. ACE

Third-generation cephalosporins (cefotaxime, ceftazidime and ceftriaxone) have broad-spectrum activity and are effective for treatment against most gram-negative organisms (including beta-lactamase-producing *Haemophilus influenzae*) and some gram-positive organisms (e.g. *Streptococcus pneumoniae* and *Streptococcus pyogenes*). They are less effective for *Staphylococcus aureus* infections. Their mode of action is similar to that of penicillins in that they inhibit bacterial cell wall synthesis. They are also primarily excreted by the kidney, although ceftriaxone has a dual hepatic and renal excretion route. The main side-effect of cephalosporins is possible hypersensitivity and approximately 10% of patients with known penicillin hypersensitivity are also allergic to cephalosporins.

60. ACDE

The anion gap is normally about 12 mmol/l. It is the difference between the cations (principally sodium and potassium) and the anions (principally consisting of chloride and bicarbonate ions). A rise in the gap shows the presence of an unmeasured cation or anion. In diabetic ketoacidosis this is beta-hydroxybutyrate and acetoacetate and in renal failure retained phosphate and sulphate. In proximal renal tubular acidosis the defect is one of bicarbonate loss and the anion gap remains unchanged.

Paper 5

1. **Fetal haemoglobin (HbF):**
   A. consists of two beta (2b) and two gamma (2c) globin chains.
   B. accounts for over 95% of the total haemoglobin at term.
   C. has less affinity for oxygen than haemoglobin A (HbA).
   D. is affected in alpha-thalassaemia.
   E. is undetectable by 6 months of age.

2. **It is considered safe to breast feed when the mother is on the following drugs:**
   A. amiodarone.
   B. warfarin.
   C. ciprofloxacin.
   D. rifampicin.
   E. sodium valproate.

3. **The following statements regarding coarctation of the aorta are correct:**
   A. coarctation of the aorta is associated with a bicuspid aortic valve in more than 50% of cases.
   B. when preductal, coarctation of the aorta is frequently associated with other cardiac defects.
   C. coarctation of the aorta is suggested by a pressure difference of 10–15 mmHg between the upper and lower limbs.
   D. coarctation of the aorta may present in the neonatal period with acute collapse, acidosis and renal failure.
   E. hypertension may occur following surgical repair.

1. **D**

   Fetal haemoglobin (HbF) consists of two alpha and two gamma globin chains. It is the predominant haemoglobin during fetal life and production begins to decline from about 32 weeks gestation. At 32–34 weeks approximately 90% of total haemoglobin is fetal and 10% adult (HbA). By term the proportion of HbF has fallen to approximately 70–80%, and this declines further to about 1% by 6 months of age. HbF has a greater affinity for oxygen because of its lesser affinity with 2,3-diphosphoglycerate. The alpha-thalassaemias result from deletions of the four genes coding for alpha-globin chain production. As alpha-globin chains are common to both fetal and adult haemoglobin, homozygous forms of alpha-thalassaemia can present either in *utero* or in the perinatal period.

2. **BDE**

   Amiodarone is present in the milk in significant amounts and should be avoided. Warfarin is safe but phenindione should be avoided. High amounts of ciprofloxacin appear in the milk so should be avoided. Rifampicin and sodium valproate are excreted in breast milk in too small quantities to be harmful.

3. **ABDE**

   Coarctation of the aorta (CoA) has a slight male preponderance and accounts for about 8% of all congenital heart disease. The most commonly affected part of the aorta is in the upper thoracic section. Preductal CoA is associated with other cardiac defects in about 40% of cases (ventricular septal defect, patent ductus arteriosus, transposition of the great arteries). These children become symptomatic in very early life. Postductal CoA is usually an isolated defect and usually does not produce symptoms in infancy. A blood pressure gradient of > 20 mmHg suggests CoA. Severe cases classically present at around 10 days of age with acute collapse, acidosis and renal failure. Prompt diagnosis and aggressive treatment is necessary. Hypertension may persist long term, even after successful repair of the CoA.

4. **The following statements regarding Wilson's disease are correct:**
   A. low caeruloplasmin levels are diagnostic of Wilson's disease.
   B. Wilson's disease can present as a deterioration in school performance.
   C. colchicine challenge is a useful diagnostic test.
   D. total serum copper levels are always high.
   E. siblings of a child with this condition have a 1 in 4 chance of having Wilson's disease.

5. **The following occur more commonly in infants of opiate-abusing mothers:**
   A. intrauterine growth retardation.
   B. birth asphyxia.
   C. increased metabolic rate.
   D. cerebral infarction.
   E. sudden infant death syndrome (SIDS).

6. **The following are recognized features of congenital hypothyroidism:**
   A. thyroid-stimulating hormone (TSH) level of 5 mU/l.
   B. goitre.
   C. pretibial myxoedema.
   D. inguinal hernia.
   E. prolonged jaundice.

4. **BE**

   Wilson's disease is inherited as an autosomal recessive condition. It is essential that asymptomatic siblings and cousins of children with the condition are fully investigated. Although most children with Wilson's disease have a low caeruloplasmin level, levels can be normal in between 4 and 20% of patients. Low values can also be found in heterozygotes for the condition as well as in nephrotic syndrome, severe malabsorption, fulminant hepatitis, chronic active hepatitis and tyrosinaemia. The pathognomonic sign of Wilson's disease is the presence of a Kayser-Fleischer ring which can be seen on slit lamp examination. As well as hepatic manifestations of the disease, Wilson's disease can present with neurological or psychological symptoms. Urinary copper excretion, pre- and post-penicillamine challenge, should be measured in any patient with Kayser-Fleischer rings. Total serum copper can be normal, high or low.

5. **ACE**

   Infants of opiate-abusing mothers are more likely to be small for gestational age. It is uncertain whether this is due to a direct effect of the drug or, more likely, due to compromised maternal nutrition associated with the chaotic lifestyle. Opiate withdrawal in the infant leads to an increased metabolic rate. The incidence of SIDS is significantly higher in infants of opiate abusers.

6. **BE**

   Features of congenital hypothyroidism:

   > poor feeding
   > hypotonia
   > lethargy
   > prolonged jaundice
   > large tongue
   > hoarse cry
   > constipation
   > umbilical hernia
   > goitre
   > TSH > 10 mU/l (usually > 50 mU/l)
   > T4 < 10 pmol/l.

7. **Measles, mumps and rubella vaccine (MMR) is contraindicated:**
   A. in children with a fever at the time of vaccination.
   B. in children with a previous anaphylactic reaction to egg.
   C. in children with a previous measles infection.
   D. during viral upper respiratory tract infections.
   E. during treatment with high-dose systemic steroids.

8. **These epidemiological terms are correct:**
   A. incidence is the number of new cases occurring in a specified period.
   B. a very low birth-weight baby has a birth weight of less than 1500 g.
   C. standardized mortality rate (SMR) compares a mortality that occurred in a designated group with that of a standard population.
   D. validity is a measure of the capacity of a test to give a true positive.
   E. secondary attack rate is the number of new cases of a disease arising within one incubation period after the primary case(s).

9. **The following drugs decrease carbamazepine levels in the blood:**
   A. phenytoin.
   B. phenobarbitone.
   C. sodium valproate.
   D. erythromycin.
   E. isoniazid.

10. **In protein-energy malnutrition in children:**
    A. linear growth slows.
    B. weight to height ratio is usually increased.
    C. growth hormone levels are reduced.
    D. oedema is common in marasmic cases.
    E. fatty changes occur in the liver.

7. **ABE**

   Contraindications to MMR vaccine include treatment with high-dose corticosteroids and other immunosuppressive drugs, malignancy, pregnancy, a history of anaphylaxis due to any cause and recent immunoglobulin administration (within 3 months). It is also contraindicated in children with immuno-deficiency states. A non-febrile upper respiratory tract infection is not a contraindication for vaccination. Previous infection with measles, mumps or rubella is not a contraindication to vaccination with MMR.

8. **ABCE**

   SMR equals observed deaths divided by expected deaths multiplied by 100. Validity is a measure of the capacity of a test to give a true result. Secondary attack rate is equal to the number of derived infections divided by the number of susceptible persons in the group at risk.

9. **AB**

   Phenytoin and phenobarbitone induce liver enzymes and reduce the level of carbamazepine. Sodium valproate, erythromycin and isoniazid inhibit hepatic enzymes and therefore increase carbamazepine levels.

10. **AE**

    Protein-energy malnutrition (PEM) exists in various forms depending on the relative proportion of protein and calorie deficiency. Marasmus, the most common form, is secondary to calorie deficiency. Kwashiorkor leads to marked oedema as a result of severe protein malnutrition. PEM leads to a decreased weight to height ratio, although linear growth does slow down. Insulin levels are low, whereas levels of growth hormone, cortisol and thyroxine are elevated leading to decreased glucose utilization by tissues. In Kwashiorkor, the overall protein deficiency leads to decreased hepatic synthesis of lipoproteins, which results in fatty changes in the liver.

11. **The following are recognized in myasthenia gravis:**
    A. ophthalmoplegia.
    B. symptoms worse first thing in the morning.
    C. antibodies to the acetylcholine receptor.
    D. abnormal electromyograph.
    E. Elevated creatine phosphokinase.

12. **These associations are correct:**
    A. anisocytosis — defective erythropoiesis.
    B. spherocytosis — acquired haemolytic anaemia.
    C. normoblasts — acute leukaemia.
    D. increased mean corpuscular volume — aplastic anaemia.
    E. lymphocytosis — bordetella pertussis.

13. **The following statements regarding gastroenteritis in children are correct:**
    A. prolonged diarrhoea and failure to recover from gastro-enteritis is rarely due to an enzyme deficiency.
    B. most infants can be managed conservatively with enteral fluids.
    C. it is important to exclude all milk from the diet for a short period.
    D. rapid rehydration is necessary in hypernatraemic dehydration in order to restore the serum sodium to normal.
    E. enterotoxins contribute to diarrhoea by stimulating fluid secretion by decreasing activity of intestinal adenyl cyclase.

11. **ACD**

Myasthenia gravis may present in older children with ophthal-moplegia, ptosis and diplopia or in neonates of mothers with the disease. The neonatal form leads to transient hypotonia and feeding difficulties and may last up to 2–3 months. Symptoms are worse later on in the day. Electromyography shows gradually decreasing response to repeated nerve stimulation. Antibodies to the acetylcholine receptor can be demonstrated and intravenous edrophonium chloride can be used to confirm the diagnosis (Tensilon test).

12. **ABCDE**

Haematological finding	Cause/condition
Anisocytosis/poikilocytosis	Any anaemia
Spherocytosis	Hereditary spherocytosis, acquired haemolytic anaemia
Normoblastosis	Normal neonate, bone marrow infiltration: acute leukaemia, acute anaemia, anoxia
Macrocytosis (increased mean corpuscular volume)	Folate deficiency, vitamin B_{12} deficiency, aplastic anaemia, haemolytic anaemia, liver disease, leukaemia, cytotoxic drug therapy
Lymphocytosis	Infectious mononucleosis, rubella, *Bordetella pertussis*, acute infectious lymphocytosis, hepatitis, cytomegalovirus, tuberculosis, toxoplasmosis, brucellosis, thyrotoxicosis.

13. **B**

Lactose intolerance is a common sequel of gastroenteritis resulting from temporary deficiency of the disaccharidase, lactase, secondary to diffuse mucosal damage. Even with mild to moderate dehydration most infants can be managed with enteral fluids. Milk does not need to be excluded. Rapid reduction in the serum sodium in hypernatraemic dehydration is dangerous and may produce seizures. Enterotoxins increase adenyl cyclase activity and increases enterocyte cyclic AMP. This results in an efflux of salt and water into the intestinal lumen.

14. **The mucous membranes may be affected in the following conditions:**
    A. dermatitis herpetiformis.
    B. lichen planus.
    C. pityriasis versicolor.
    D. Kawasaki's disease.
    E. Stevens-Johnson syndrome.

15. **A 7-year-old child with pneumonia is found to have a $PaCO_2$ of 8 kPa. The following statements are correct:**
    A. cerebral perfusion will be decreased.
    B. there will be an increased secretion of bicarbonate ions in the urine.
    C. the oxygen dissociation curve will be shifted to the left.
    D. the concentration of hydrogen ions in the plasma will be increased.
    E. the pH of the plasma will inevitably be less than normal.

16. **Antibodies cross the placenta causing disease in the fetus/neonate in the following conditions:**
    A. dystrophica myotonica.
    B. diabetes insipidus.
    C. hyperthyroidism.
    D. myasthenia gravis.
    E. idiopathic thrombocytopenic purpura.

14. **ABDE**

Mucous membranes (MM) may be affected by developmental disorders, infection, acute and chronic skin conditions, genodermatosis, benign and malignant tumours. Dermatitis herpetiformis occasionally has MM involvement, Lichen planus commonly affects the MM. Other important conditions affecting the MM are: Kawasaki's disease, Stevens-Johnson syndrome, toxic shock syndrome, mucocutaneous candidiasis and mucocutaneous leishmaniasis. Some specific conditions of the MM include: Fordyce disease (aberrant sebaceous glands), geographic tongue, cheilitis, oral thrush and aphthous stomatitis.

15. **All False**

In conditions where hypercarbia is present there is an increase in cerebral blood flow. This can lead to increased intracranial pressure and result in cerebral oedema. The kidneys respond to an increase in $PaCO_2$ by excreting hydrogen ions and conserving sodium bicarbonate. For this reason an acid urine will be present. If a raised $PaCO_2$ has been present for some time a fully compensated respiratory acidosis may occur resulting in a normal plasma pH. In conditions where a respiratory acidosis is present, the oxygen dissociation curve will move to the right thus decreasing the affinity of haemoglobin for oxygen (see Question 14, Paper 4).

16. **CDE**

Infants born to mothers with dystrophica myotonica are likely to be affected with the condition but not as a result of antibody transfer. Mothers who have been thyrotoxic will have circulating IgG antibodies that may affect the neonate. About 10% of infants born to mothers with myasthenia gravis are affected by an IgG antibody. Autoimmune thrombocytopenia occurs in neonates of mothers who suffer from idiopathic thrombocytopenic purpura. Mothers who are Zw^b antigen negative can produce an IgG antibody to Zw^a antigen (present in 98% population). This can cause an isoimmune neonatal thrombocytopenia.

17. **Petit mal epilepsy:**
    A. may be precipitated by hyperventilation.
    B. is characterized by burst suppression on an EEG.
    C. carries a poor prognosis.
    D. rarely has a family history.
    E. commonly occurs in infants.

18. **A baby is born to a mother who is known to be HIV positive. The following tests confirm that the infant is infected:**
    A. the presence of HIV antibody.
    B. HIV virus culture positive on two separate occasions.
    C. positive polymerase chain reaction (PCR) on two separate occasions.
    D. CD4:CD8 ratio <1.
    E. p24 antigenaemia on two separate occasions.

19. **Major criteria for the diagnosis of acute rheumatic fever include:**
    A. arthralgia.
    B. fever.
    C. erythema marginatum.
    D. chorea.
    E. 1st degree heart block.

17. **A**

Hyperventilation produces both clinical features (absences) and EEG features of petit mal. The EEG in a child with petit mal epilepsy typically shows a 3 Hz spike and wave pattern. Petit mal epilepsy becomes less of a problem in teenagers and medication may be stopped. A strong family history of children suffering from petit mal epilepsy is often found. The most commonly affected age group is between 5 and 10 years of age.

18. **BCE**

All babies born to HIV antibody positive mothers will also be antibody positive as a result of placental transfer. Persistence of the HIV antibody beyond 18 months when measured on two separate occasions is diagnostic of HIV infection. In a newborn infant born to an HIV infected mother, diagnosis can be made by detection of the antigen in culture, the presence of the HIV genome on PCR, or the presence of p24 antigen. These need to be measured on two separate occasions at least 2 weeks apart for the diagnosis to be made. The CD4:CD8 ratio is too variable in newborn infants to be used as a single diagnostic test for HIV infection.

19. **CD**

Major criteria for rheumatic fever are:

   carditis
   flitting polyarthritis
   erythema marginatum
   subcutaneous nodules
   chorea.

Minor criteria include:

   fever
   arthralgia
   raised erythrocyte sedimentation rate
   raised antistreptolysin O titre
   1st degree heart block
   raised white cell count
   raised c-reactive protein
   previous acute rheumatic fever.

20. **The following statements regarding encopresis are correct:**
    A. children with this condition are usually constipated.
    B. stressful life events may precipitate the condition.
    C. clinical depression is more common in children with encopresis than in the normal population.
    D. spinal cord lesions can present with encopresis.
    E. family psychotherapy may be indicated.

21. **Surfactant production:**
    A. takes place in type 1 pneumocytes.
    B. can be detected at 20 weeks gestation.
    C. is decreased by maternal corticosteroid administration.
    D. is increased by intrauterine growth retardation (IUGR).
    E. is decreased by maternal opiate abuse.

22. **A normal 4 year old would be expected to be able to:**
    A. catch a ball.
    B. draw a circle.
    C. count to 10.
    D. tell you his/her name and address.
    E. get dressed alone.

23. **Features of pyloric stenosis include:**
    A. hyperchloraemic hypokalaemic metabolic alkalosis.
    B. bile-stained vomiting.
    C. a low urinary pH.
    D. a greater incidence in boys than girls.
    E. an association with Down's syndrome.

24. **The following drugs may be safely used in renal failure:**
    A. salbutamol.
    B. gentamicin.
    C. metolazone.
    D. frusemide.
    E. nitrofurantoin.

20. BCDE

Encopresis is defined as the passage of normal stools in abnormal places. Children with encopresis are not usually constipated. In most cases organic causes for the problem can be excluded. Another important differential diagnosis for encopresis is Crohn's disease. Family and/or individual psychotherapy may help in the treatment of the condition.

21. BD

Surfactant is produced by type 2 pneumocytes. Although small amounts may be detected as early as 20 weeks gestation, physiologically significant quantities may not be produced until 30–32 weeks. Surfactant production may be accelerated by several maternally ingested substances including glucocorticoids and opiates. IUGR and other causes of intrauterine 'stress' may also enhance production of surfactant.

22. ABCDE

See Question 17, Paper 1.

23. CD

The metabolic abnormality in pyloric stenosis is a hypochloraemic hypokalaemic metabolic alkalosis caused by loss of potassium, chloride and sodium. The urine is paradoxically acidic as the kidneys attempt to reabsorb potassium in the urine in exchange for hydrogen ions in the blood.

24. ABCD

Salbutamol is useful in the emergency treatment of acute hyperkalaemia. Gentamicin can be used in renal failure as long as plasma concentrations are monitored carefully and dosage reduced. The thiazide diuretics should be avoided in renal failure except for metolazone which remains effective. There is a risk of excessive diuresis with metolazone therapy. Nitrofurantoin accumulates in renal failure and causes a peripheral neuropathy.

25. **The following are causes of secondary lactose intolerance in infancy:**
    A. rotavirus infection.
    B. giardiasis.
    C. coeliac disease.
    D. cow's milk protein intolerance.
    E. soya protein intolerance.

26. **Causes of splenomegaly in childhood include:**
    A. Gaucher's disease.
    B. typhoid.
    C. acute meningococcal septicaemia.
    D. systemic lupus erythematosus (SLE).
    E. galactosaemia.

27. **The following are indications for renal tract ultrasound in the newborn period:**
    A. failure to pass urine during the first 12 hours of life.
    B. systolic blood pressure of 65 mmHg in a term infant.
    C. hypospadius.
    D. imperforate anus.
    E. antenatal ultrasound diagnosis of unilateral hydronephrosis.

28. **In the development of the fetus the following statements are true:**
    A. the epithelial lining of the wall of the gut is derived from the ectoderm layer.
    B. monozygotic twins always share the same placenta.
    C. the heart is derived from the mesoderm layer.
    D. the epididymis is derived from the paramesonephric duct.
    E. the thyroid gland is derived from the 3rd pharyngeal pouch.

25. **ABCDE**

Disaccharidase deficiency in infancy and early childhood is most commonly secondary to small bowel mucosal damage after gastroenteritis. Other possible causes of mucosal damage include coeliac disease, giardiasis, cow's milk protein intolerance and other milk protein intolerance. Primary lactase intolerance is rare but may present early in white people or after 2–3 years in black people.

26. **ABDE**

There are many causes of splenomegaly, including: haemolytic anaemias, haemoglobinopathies, thalassaemias, typhoid, endocarditis, infectious mononucleosis, malaria, toxoplasmosis, portal or splenic vein obstruction, cirrhosis, chronic heart failure, Niemann-Pick disease, Gaucher's disease, leukaemia, lymphoma (Hodgkins' and non-Hodgkins), angiomas, rheumatoid arthritis and SLE.

27. **CDE**

It has been estimated that approximately 92% of normal neonates pass urine by 24 hours of life. An acceptable systolic blood pressure in a term infant on day 1 is between approximately 55–80 mmHg. Any genital, anal or perineal anomaly may be associated with abnormalities of the renal tract and therefore an ultrasound scan should be carried out to exclude these. All antenatally diagnosed anomalies of the renal tract should be followed-up with a postnatal ultrasound scan.

28. **C**

The gastrointestinal tract is the main organ system derived from the endoderm layer. The mesoderm layer gives rise to the cardiovascular system and the ectoderm layer gives rise to the central and peripheral nervous systems. Monozygotic twins can share a placenta depending on the point at which the two-stage zygote splits. They may share a common amniotic sac or chorionic cavity again depending on the stage of zygote splitting. However, monozygotic twins may have separate placentas, amniotic sacs and chorionic cavities. The epididymis is derived from the mesonephric duct and the female genitourinary tract is derived from the paramesonephric ducts. The parathyroid gland is derived from the 3rd pharyngeal pouch.

29. In Reye syndrome:
A. there is a strong association with varicella infection.
B. a metabolic alkalosis is often present.
C. raised ammonia levels in the blood is diagnostic.
D. hypoglycaemia is always present.
E. the treatment of choice is liver transplantation.

30. In human neurons:
A. myelin sheaths extend across the nodes of Ranvier.
B. unmyelinated fibres have faster conduction.
C. sodium ion influx occurs during the action potential.
D. the action potential increases with increased stimulation.
E. increased extracellular calcium leads to increased neuronal excitability.

31. Small-for-gestational-age infants are more likely than appropriate-for-gestational-age infants to have:
A. hypoglycaemia.
B. hypocalcaemia.
C. respiratory distress syndrome.
D. congenital malformations.
E. persistent fetal circulation.

32. The second heart sound:
A. splitting is decreased during inspiration.
B. splitting is fixed in patients with atrial septal defect (ASD).
C. is usually single in tetralogy of Fallot.
D. is inaudible in pulmonary hypertension.
E. the aortic component normally occurs before the pulmonary component.

29. A

Reye syndrome is preceded by varicella infection in 5–7% of cases. There is a probable association with aspirin ingestion. A metabolic acidosis is often present together with raised ammonia levels. Raised ammonia levels are also seen in urea cycle defects as well as organic acidaemias. Hypoglycaemia is often seen in younger children but less so in older children. The characteristic lesion in Reye syndrome is that of fatty infiltration of the liver. Treatment of choice is conservative therapy, which aims to reduce raised intracranial pressure resulting from the associated encephalopathy.

30. C

Myelin sheaths are interrupted by the nodes of Ranvier allowing depolarization to jump from one node to another and increase conduction velocity. This is called saltatory conduction and it allows a more than 50-fold increase in conduction speed in myelinated fibres. The action potential occurs as a result of sodium ion influx and potassium efflux from the neuron and is an 'all or none' phenomenon. Decreased extracellular calcium concentration leads to a lowering of the threshold for neuronal depolarization and thereby increases nerve cell excitability.

31. ACE

Small for gestational age fetuses are more likely than normal newborn infants to encounter several problems in the neonatal period. These include: hypothermia, hypoglycaemia due to reduced glycogen stores, impaired gluconeogenesis and relative hyperinsulinism, hyperglycaemia, respiratory difficulties (meconium aspiration and chest infections), polycythaemia and persistent fetal circulation.

32. BCE

The normal splitting of the second heart sound (A2 before P2) is increased during inspiration, widely split and fixed in patients with an ASD, is usually single in tetralogy of Fallot and is loud in pulmonary hypertension.

33. **A five-year-old child presents with a high swinging fever. A diagnosis of systemic onset juvenile chronic arthritis (JCA) is more likely if the following features are present:**
    A. the child is female.
    B. HLA studies show that the child is HLA-B27.
    C. the child is rheumatoid factor positive.
    D. iridocyclitis is present.
    E. hepatospenomegaly is present.

34. **In normal puberty:**
    A. levels of luteinizing hormone (LH) rise before follicle-stimulating hormone (FSH) in girls.
    B. development of pubic hair is the first sign of puberty in girls.
    C. an increase in testes occurs before increase in penile size in boys.
    D. menarche over the age of 15 years occurs in 20% of girls.
    E. menarche usually coincides with the peak of the height velocity curve seen during the puberty-associated growth spurt.

35. **A 5-year-old boy refuses to go to school. The following statements regarding school phobia are correct:**
    A. it is more common in boys than girls.
    B. it is associated with a low IQ.
    C. somatic complaints often accompany the phobia.
    D. truancy is common in children who have school refusal.
    E. school phobia has a better prognosis in early childhood than in adolescence.

36. **Criteria for the diagnosis of brain stem death include:**
    A. a flat EEG.
    B. two doctors to make a diagnosis of brain stem death.
    C. no ventilatory response to hypoxia.
    D. absent corneal reflexes.
    E. the absence of hypothermia.

33. E

Systemic onset JCA is typified by a persistent, high swinging fever, a 'rheumatoid' rash, hepatosplenomegaly, lymphadeno- pathy and pleuritis. It has an equal sex distribution. HLA associations with the condition are not yet known. HLA-B27 is seen in about 90% of children seen with juvenile ankylosing spondylitis. Children with systemic onset JCA are rheumatoid factor negative and do not develop iridocyclitis. In pauciarti- cular JCA up to 50% of those who are antinuclear factor positive will develop chronic iridocyclitis.

34. C

Levels of oestriol increase with advancing sexual maturation along with levels of FSH. LH levels do not increase until secondary sexual characteristics are well developed. In girls the first sign of puberty is breast bud development. Testicular enlargement is the first sign of puberty in boys. Age range for menarche is 11.0–15.0 years. Less than 3% will have menarche after 15 years. Menarche is associated with the deceleration phase of the height velocity curve seen in puberty.

35. CE

In truancy, children leave home but do not arrive at school or leave early. It is commonly associated with a low IQ and is more common in boys than girls, unlike school phobia which has an equal sex ratio. Often in children suffering from school phobia there are functional symptoms present such as abdominal pain or headaches. The condition carries a better prognosis if treated and recognized at an earlier age.

36. BDE

Brain stem death should be diagnosed by two doctors. There are three steps to making a diagnosis of brain stem death. Firstly the patient must be unresponsive on a ventilator with a clear cause of coma. Secondly, all potential causes of reversible coma must be excluded. These include drug depression of the central nervous system, metabolic or endocrine disturbances or primary hypother- mia. Thirdly, brain stem areflexia and persistent apnoea must be present. For brain stem areflexia to be present there must be no pupillary response to light, no corneal reflex, no vestibulo-occular reflex, no gag reflex and no response to stimulation of any somatic area. Apnoea is tested by allowing the $PaCO_2$ to rise above 6.66 kPa with no ventilatory response within 10 minutes.

37. **The following statements are correct:**
   A. in a type 2 error, the null hypothesis is falsely rejected.
   B. the power of a study is related to the size of the sample.
   C. contingency tables compare proportions arising from categorical data.
   D. a chi-squared distribution can only have positive values.
   E. relative risks can be calculated from retrospective data.

38. **It is advised by the Department of Health that children who are HIV positive and who have symptoms of AIDS can receive the following vaccines:**
   A. MMR.
   B. Hib.
   C. pertussis.
   D. oral typhoid.
   E. BCG.

39. **The following statements are true regarding the urinary tract in early life:**
   A. all children under the age of 5 years who have a proven urinary tract infection (UTI) should have a micturating cystogram.
   B. UTIs are more common in newborn boys than girls.
   C. vesico-ureteric reflux is the cause of renal failure in up to 20% of children.
   D. pulmonary hypoplasia is associated with the presence of posterior urethral valves.
   E. ultrasonography is the investigation of choice in the diagnosis of renal scarring.

37. **BCD**

In a type 1 error, a significant result is obtained when the null hypothesis is correct. In other words it is a false-positive. In a type 2 error, a significant result is present when the null hypothesis has been rejected. In other words a false-negative is obtained. The power of a study is the probability that a study of a given size will detect a significant difference in the study group. The power is dependent on the size of the sample, the standard deviation of the difference that is being investigated and the level of significance that is being sought. A large sample size, a small standard deviation and a high level of significance all increase the power of a study. In categorical data there is only possible outcomes for data, e.g., the presence or absence of a disease or a physical sign. Relative risks can only be calculated from prospective studies. Odds ratios can be estimated from retrospective data.

38. **ABC**

The Department of Health has advised that HIV positive patients with or without symptoms can receive the following: live vaccines: measles, MMR, mumps, poliomyelitis, rubella. Inactivated vaccines: cholera, diphtheria, Hib, hepatitis A, hepatitis B, influenza, meningococcal, pertussis, pneumococcal, poliomyelitis, tetanus, typhoid (injection). HIV positive patients should not receive: BCG, yellow fever, oral typhoid vaccines.

39. **BCD**

Although it is not accepted by all paediatricians, most would agree that a micturating cystourethrogram is indicated in any child with a proven UTI under the age of 1 year. Radio-nucleotide imaging techniques such as the dimercaptosuccinic acid (DMSA) scan are the most accurate way of detecting renal scarring.

40. A 5-year-old child presents with a purpuric rash. She is otherwise completely well. Her platelet count is 8 × 10⁹/l. The rest of the blood count is normal. After a bone marrow biopsy a diagnosis of idiopathic thrombocytopenic purpura (ITP) is made. The following statements are correct:
   A. a bone marrow biopsy should be performed in all cases of suspected ITP.
   B. the bone marrow will show a suppression of megakaryocyte activity.
   C. the bleeding time will be increased.
   D. there is an 80% chance that the child will spontaneously recover within 1 year.
   E. intravenous gammaglobulin shortens the course of the disease.

41. In infections caused by the Epstein-Barr virus (EBV):
   A. only T cells are infected.
   B. lymphoproliferative disease can be seen following an infection.
   C. Burkitt's lymphoma can develop as the result of being infected.
   D. a Coombs' positive haemolytic anaemia can develop as the result of being infected.
   E. the atypical cells found in the peripheral blood film in infectious mononucleosis are T cells.

42. The following drugs are paired with recognized side-effects:
   A. salbutamol   – hyperkalaemia.
   B. indomethacin   – decreased urine output.
   C. aminophylline   – increased urine output.
   D. frusemide   – decreased urinary calcium excretion.
   E. hydrochlorothiazide – hypoglycaemia.

40. ACDE

All children who present with suspected ITP should have a bone marrow biopsy performed even if examination of the child is normal apart from the purpuric rash. Occult aplastic or infiltrative processes may be missed. The bone marrow in ITP has increased or normal numbers of megakaryocytes. The disease process is due to destruction of platelets by antiplatelet IgG which can appear following a viral infection. Intravenous gammaglobulin at a dose of 400 mg/kg/day for 5 days may shorten the course of the disease, probably by interfering with the function of the antiplatelet IgG. A response may be seen within 48 hours of usage. Most children spontaneously recover within 6 months of the onset of the illness. Some experience chronic problems which may respond to a splenectomy.

41. BCDE

The Epstein-Barr virus (EBV) infects solely B cells although the atypical cells seen in infectious mononucleosis are T cells. EBV has a role in lymphoproliferative disease that is commonly seen in children after transplantation who are on immunosuppressive treatment. When trying to diagnose EBV infection, the first serum marker to appear is the antibody to anti-viral capsid antigen. The last marker to appear is the antibody to the Epstein-Barr nuclear antigen. Acyclovir may be used in treatment. Numerous abnormal antibodies are found in children infected with EBV; this may result in a Coombs' positive haemolytic anaemia.

42. BC

Salbutamol lowers serum potassium and may lead to hypokalaemia. Indomethacin is a powerful renal vasoconstrictive agent and therefore decreases urine output by decreasing glomerular filtration rate. Theophyllines have weak diuretic properties. Frusemide increases urinary calcium excretion and may be useful in severe hypercalcaemia. Thiazide diuretics inhibit pancreatic insulin release and may therefore cause hyperglycaemia.

43. Retinitis pigmentosa can be found in the following conditions:
A. Tay-Sachs' disease.
B. Lawrence-Moon-Biedel syndrome.
C. Krabbe disease.
D. Abetalipoproteinaemia.
E. Refsum's disease.

44. Cardiomyopathy can be a feature of:
A. Friedreich's ataxia.
B. Marfan's syndrome.
C. neurofibromatosis.
D. Duchenne muscular dystrophy.
E. Rubenstein-Taybi syndrome.

45. In cystic fibrosis (CF):
A. presentation may be with a congenital pneumonia.
B. the gene responsible for CF is on the long arm of chromosome 7.
C. the gene mutation delta F501 occurs in about 75% of cases.
D. a sweat test with 50 mmol/l of sodium is diagnostic.
E. meconium ileus accounts for about 20% of presentations.

46. Changes in circulation that normally occur after birth:
A. are partly caused by a rise in circulating prostaglandin levels.
B. may normally lead to a left to right shunt across the ductus arteriosus persisting for up to 24 hours.
C. may be delayed by respiratory distress syndrome (RDS).
D. may be delayed by cyanotic congenital heart disease.
E. may be delayed by nitric oxide.

43. BDE

Retinitis pigmentosa is a progressive degeneration of the retina with characteristic changes in pigment and a degree of optic atrophy. As well as being a disease entity in its own right it is seen in many other conditions leading to increasing visual impairment. Lawrence-Moon-Biedel syndrome is the association of hypothalamic and pituitary dysfunction with mental retardation, post-axial polydactyly, renal problems and retinitis pigmentosa. Refsum's disease is diagnosed by increased phytanic acid in the serum. It is inherited as an autosomal recessive trait and presents with failing vision as a result of retinitis pigmentosa, weakness and unsteady gait.

44. AD

In both Friedreich's ataxia and Duchenne muscular dystrophy, the associated cardiomyopathy can be the terminal event in the illnesses. Marfan's syndrome is associated with aortic dilatation and dissecting aortic aneurysm. Neurofibromatosis is associated with coarctation of the aorta, pulmonary stenosis and phaeo-chromocytoma.

45. ABE

CF is the most common cause of chronic suppurative lung disease in children and adolescents in the UK. It is an autosomal recessive condition with a population carrier rate of 1 in 25. About 1 infant in 2500 is affected. The CF gene is located on the long arm of chromosome 7. The most common mutating allele is delta F508, which accounts for 75–85% cases in the UK. The basic defect appears to be the chloride transmembrane regulator protein. The clinical and diagnostic features arise from effects on the exocrine glandular system. The respiratory and gastrointestinal tracts are mainly affected with increasing problems as the child gets older. The sweat test is still the gold standard for routine diagnosis. Pilocarpine iontophoresis is used and the test is diagnostic if the sweat sodium is > 70 mmol/l from an adequate sample (>100 mg sweat). Congenital pneumonia and meconium ileus should always suggest CF as a possible diagnosis.

46. BCD

It is important to understand the anatomy of the fetal circulation and the physiological changes that occur around the time of birth. Also see Question 9, Paper 3.

47. **The following statements regarding tumour necrosis factor (TNF) are correct:**
    A. TNF is secreted by neutrophils.
    B. TNF release causes pyrexia.
    C. TNF activates macrophages.
    D. TNF is present in tubercule granulomas.
    E. TNF is a cytokine.

48. **A newborn infant presents with convulsions at 4 hours of age. The following diagnoses should be considered:**
    A. hypoglycaemia.
    B. hypomagnesaemia.
    C. myotonic dystrophica.
    D. pyridoxine deficiency.
    E. hereditary fructose intolerance.

49. **In Turner's syndrome:**
    A. most affected fetuses will abort in early pregnancy.
    B. growth hormone has no effect on final adult height.
    C. pulmonary stenosis commonly occurs.
    D. horseshoe kidney occurs in about 50% of cases.
    E. expected IQ is about 80.

47. BCDE

TNF is secreted by macrophages and lymphocytes. It enhances the microbicidal activity of macrophages. TNF also induces null killer cells to release interferon, which further increases the bacteriocidal activity of macrophages. TNF release may also be harmful in that there is evidence that it has a role in the formation of granulomas in tuberculosis.

48. ABDE

The list of the differential diagnoses of a convulsion within the first 4 hours of life must include: sepsis (especially meningitis), intracranial haemorrhage, subdural haemorrhage, asphyxia, hypocalcaemia, hypomagnesaemia, hyponatraemia, drug withdrawal, and inborn errors of metabolism. Pyridoxine deficiency is rare but should be considered if there is no obvious cause for the fitting. Infants usually will respond to 100 mg of pyridoxine given intravenously. Infants with dystrophica myotonica present with hypotonia. Convulsions may occur if milk feeds containing fructose or sucrose are given to an infant with hereditary fructose intolerance.

49. AD

Turner's syndrome (45,X) occurs in about 1 in 3000 live births; 95% of all 45,XO conceptions are aborted. Recombinant human growth hormone has been given for the short stature and has a modest effect on final height. Coarctation of the aorta occurs in about 15% of cases, isolated non-stenotic bicuspid valve has been detected in about one-third of cases, and horseshoe kidney in 50% of cases. IQ is usually normal.

50. **Conditions associated with an increased risk of malignant neoplasia during childhood include:**
    A. aniridia.
    B. ataxia telangiectasia.
    C. Fanconi's anaemia.
    D. 13q- syndrome.
    E. Peutz-Jegher's syndrome.

51. **The following statements regarding glomerular disease are correct:**
    A. antigen–antibody immune complexes activate complement via the alternative pathway.
    B. crescent formation can be present in Bowman's space.
    C. Berger's disease has only IgA mesangial deposits.
    D. children aged from 2 to 3 years are most commonly affected by the post streptococcal glomerulonephritis.
    E. diffuse thickening of the glomerular basement membrane is the most common cause of nephrotic syndrome in adults.

52. **The following statements are correct:**
    A. the ovulation age is the same as the menstrual age.
    B. the embryonic stage lasts until the end of the 8th week of gestation.
    C. the maxillary process fuses with the lateral nasal folds at about 7 weeks.
    D. mesenchyme from the 2nd pharyngeal arch forms the facial muscles.
    E. failure of fusion of the palatal processes results in a cleft lip.

50. **ABCD**
Aniridia (sporadic) along with hemihypertrophy, renal dysplasia and Beckwith-Wiedemann syndrome are all associated with an increased incidence of Wilms' tumour. Ataxia telangiectasia is associated with an increased incidence of lymphoma and leukaemia. Fanconi's anaemia is also associated with an increased risk of developing leukaemias as well as hepatomas. 13q- syndrome is associated with an increased risk of developing a retinoblastoma. Other important associations include: xeroderma pigmentosa – skin cancer; congenital X-linked immunodeficiency and severe combined immunodeficiency disease – lymphoma and leukaemia; familial IgM deficiency and Wiskott-Aldrich syndrome – lymphoma; Down syndrome – leukaemia; 11p- syndrome – Wilms' tumour; von Hippel-Landau syndrome – phaeochromocytoma; multiple endocrine adenomatosis I – schwannoma; multiple endocrine adenomatosis II – phaeochromocytoma and thyroid carcinoma; familial polyposis – carcinoma of the colon. In Peutz-Jegher's syndrome the polyps are benign hamartomas but can undergo malignant change in adulthood.

51. **BE**
Antigen–antibody immune complexes may produce glomerular disease but via activation of the classical pathway. Crescents are the result of proliferation of parietal epithelial cells in Bowman's capsule. Berger's disease has predominantly IgA deposits but smaller amounts of IgG, IgM, C3 and properidin can be present. Post-streptococcal nephritis rarely occurs in children aged less than 3 years.

52. **BCD**
The menstrual age is 14 days more than ovulation age. The pre-embryonic stage is the first 3 weeks following fertilization. The embryonic stage is complete at the end of the 8th week. The fetal stage is from the end of the 8th week until delivery. Failure of fusion of the maxillary process and the lateral nasal folds at about 7 weeks results in a cleft lip. Failure of fusion of the palatal processes results in a cleft palate.

53. **The following are correct associations:**

    A. microcytosis — thalassaemia trait.

    B. decreased mean corpuscular
       haemoglobin (MCH) — hypothyroidism.

    C. target cells — haemolytic anaemia.

    D. Burr cells — haemolytic uraemic
       syndrome.

    E. polychromasia — bone marrow inactivity.

54. **A child is seen in outpatients with a left-sided facial palsy with sparing of the muscles of the forehead on the affected side. The following conditions could account for this presentation:**

    A. Guillain-Barré syndrome.

    B. left-sided cerebral tumour.

    C. right-sided cerebral haemorrhage.

    D. pontine tumour.

    E. Bell's palsy.

55. **The following statements about Kawasaki's disease are correct:**

    A. thrombocytosis is commonly found in the first week of the illness.

    B. there is no associated mortality.

    C. cardiac manifestations of the disease are present in 20% of cases.

    D. high-dose aspirin protects against the formation of coronary artery aneurysms.

    E. the presence of the disease in an infant under the age of 1 year indicates a higher risk of coronary artery aneurysm formation.

53.   ABCD

Haematological finding	Causes/conditions
Microcytosis (decreased mean corpuscular volume)	Iron deficiency, thalassaemia trait
Hypochromasia (decreased MCH)	Iron deficiency, haemoglobinopathies, lead poisoning, isoniazid, juvenile arthritis, tuberculosis, uraemia, hypothyroidism, malignancy
Target cells	Haemolytic anaemia, obstructive jaundice, hypochromic anaemia
Burr cells, fragmentation (schistocytosis)	Consumptive coagulopathy (DIC), renal failure
Polychromasia	Active bone marrow.

54.   C

The child has presented with typical signs of an upper motor neuron lesion. These lesions cause weakness to the lower part of the face on the side opposite the lesion. In Guillain-Barré syndrome, pontine tumours and Bell's palsy the signs are those of a lower motor neuron lesion with weakness of all the muscles of facial expression on the same side.

55.   CE

The platelet count is normal in the first week of the illness, rises in the second and peaks in the third week. There is a mortality of 1% in Kawasaki's disease which is usually due to massive cardiac infarction as a result of coronary artery thrombosis. The cardiac manifestations of the disease in the acute phase are: myocarditis, pericarditis, valvular insufficiency and arrhythmias. Acute coronary arteritis may lead to coronary artery aneurysm formation. Whilst high-dose aspirin therapy shortens the duration of fever and reduces the inflammatory response, only intravenous immunoglobulin therapy given early in the disease reduces the rate of aneurysm formation. Factors that indicate a higher risk of aneurysm formation include: fever for more than 16 days, recurrence of fever after a 48-hour afebrile period, arrhythmias other than first-degree heart block, male sex, cardiomegaly, extreme thrombocytosis and leukocytosis.

56. **The following cause hypoglycaemia:**
    A. prednisolone.
    B. lactulose.
    C. aspirin.
    D. atenolol.
    E. alcohol.

57. **In sudden infant death syndrome (SIDS) and acute life-threatening events (ALTE) the following statements are correct:**
    A. infants should never be left to sleep lying prone.
    B. infants who have had an ALTE are not likely to die of subsequent SIDS.
    C. in infants at risk of SIDS, home monitoring with an apnoea alarm with or without pulse oximetry will prevent SIDS.
    D. ALTE may be the result of deliberate suffocation by a parent.
    E. a post-mortem examination is not always indicated in SIDS.

58. **The following are associated with macroglossia:**
    A. Down's syndrome.
    B. Beckwith-Wiedemann syndrome.
    C. hyperthyroidism.
    D. Von Gierke's disease.
    E. Hurler syndrome.

59. **The following are causes of a continuous murmur:**
    A. pulmonary hypertension.
    B. tricuspid regurgitation.
    C. patent ductus arteriosus.
    D. Blalock shunt.
    E. mitral valve prolapse.

56. **CDE**

Prolonged courses of systemic steroids may cause poor glucose tolerance and therefore increase blood sugar levels. Aspirin, beta-blockers and alcohol in high doses may lead to hypoglycaemia.

57. **D**

Despite the general recommendation that infants should sleep supine or on their side with a roll, there are medical indications (e.g. Pierre-Robin syndrome) when a baby should be allowed to sleep prone. Once an infant can roll supine to prone and vice versa, prone sleeping is thought to be safe. Following an ALTE there is an increased risk of dying from SIDS (risk between 1 and 10%). There is no evidence to suggest that apnoea alarms or pulse oximetry prevents SIDS although it may help parents through a worrying time. A post-mortem examination is always indicated because by definition the deaths are sudden and unexpected.

58. **BDE**

In Down's syndrome the oral cavity is small rather than the tongue being enlarged thus giving the impression of macroglossia. Macroglossia occurs in hypothyroidism. In Von Gierke's disease (glucose-6-phosphatase deficiency) glycogen is deposited in the tongue resulting in macroglossia. In a similar way, heparan and dermatan sulphate are deposited in the tongue in Hurler syndrome.

59. **CD**

Causes of continuous murmurs are:

> patent ductus arteriosus
> pulmonary arteriovenous fistula
> aorto-pulmonary window
> Blalock/Waterstone shunt
> venous hum.

60. **The following conditions are commonly associated with cataracts at birth:**
   A. congenital hypothyroidism.
   B. galactosaemia.
   C. congenital rubella syndrome.
   D. Lowe's syndrome.
   E. Tay-Sachs' disease.

60. BCD

In galactosaemia, cataracts are present at birth as a result of maternal derived galactose being present *in utero*. The cataracts are classically 'oil droplet' in shape and regress once the infant is put on a galactose-free diet. Congenital rubella syndrome is also associated with microphthalmos, iris hypoplasia, glaucoma, pigmentary retinopathy and optic atrophy. Lowe's syndrome is an X-linked recessive disorder associated with glaucoma, mental handicap, hypotonia and renal tubular acidosis.

Subject Index

The first number indicates the paper number. The number after the decimal point indicates the question number.

Respiratory System	Cardiovascular System	Neurology/ Development	Endocrine/ Metabolic	Therapeutics
1.01	1.03	1.17	1.04	1.07
1.22	1.19	1.21	1.13	1.08
1.53	1.29	1.45	1.27	1.15
2.22	1.37	1.47	1.30	1.24
2.46	2.08	1.55	1.32	1.35
2.56	2.28	2.06	2.26	2.21
3.10	2.47	2.10	2.30	2.23
3.21	2.53	2.16	2.54	2.45
4.09	2.57	2.25	3.24	2.52
4.47	3.11	2.42	3.31	3.06
5.45	3.33	2.49	3.47	3.25
	3.49	3.04	3.59	3.39
	4.10	3.18	4.01	4.27
	4.24	3.52	4.18	4.28
	4.36	3.53	4.50	4.40
	5.03	4.23	4.52	4.45
	5.44	4.25	5.06	4.53
	5.59	4.33	5.29	4.59
		4.54	5.43	5.02
		5.11	5.60	5.09
		5.17		5.24
		5.22		5.42
		5.36		5.56
		5.54		

Basic Sciences	Genetics	Statistics	Gastroenterology/ Hepatology	Dermatology	Neonatology
1.12	1.06	1.10	1.02	1.11	1.09
1.20	1.34	2.12	1.16	1.56	1.28
1.39	1.50	3.16	1.31	2.27	1.38
1.52	2.17	3.44	1.42	2.40	1.41
1.59	2.36	4.15	1.46	3.15	1.51
2.02	2.58	4.37	1.58	4.13	1.57
2.13	3.01	5.08	2.15	5.14	1.60
2.14	3.43	5.37	2.24		2.05
2.19	3.48		2.35		2.09
2.20	4.06		2.38		2.37
2.29	4.43		2.41		2.51
2.32	4.49		2.60		2.55
2.50	5.49		3.07		3.03
3.05	5.58		3.14		3.20
3.09			3.22		3.29
3.27			3.23		3.57
3.30			3.38		3.58
3.35			3.42		4.05
3.36			3.46		4.21
3.41			3.56		4.51
3.50			3.60		5.05
3.54			4.03		5.31
3.55			4.07		5.48
4.04			4.19		
4.08			4.39		
4.14			4.42		
4.16			4.57		
4.20			5.04		
4.31			5.10		
4.38			5.13		
4.44			5.23		
4.46			5.25		
4.56			5.26		
4.60					
5.01					
5.15					
5.21					
5.28					
5.30					
5.32					
5.34					
5.46					
5.47					
5.52					

WARNING

BY OPENING THIS SEALED PACKAGE YOU ARE AGREEING TO BECOME BOUND BY THE TERMS OF THIS LICENCE AGREEMENT which contains restrictions and limitations of liability.

IF YOU DO NOT AGREE with the terms set out here DO NOT OPEN THE PACKAGE OR BREAK THE SEAL. RETURN THE UNOPENED PACKAGE AND DISKS TO WHERE YOU BOUGHT THEM AND THE PRICE PAID WILL BE REFUNDED TO YOU.

THE MATERIAL CONTAINED IN THIS PACKAGE AND ON THE DISKS IS PROTECTED BY COPYRIGHT LAWS. HAVING PAID THE PURCHASE PRICE AND IF YOU AGREE TO THE TERMS OF THIS LICENCE BY BREAKING THE SEALS ON THE DISKS, YOU ARE HEREBY LICENSED BY WB SAUNDERS COMPANY LIMITED TO USE THE MATERIAL UPON AND SUBJECT TO THE FOLLOWING TERMS:

1. The licence is a non-exclusive right to use the written instructions, manuals and the material recorded on the disk (all of which is called the "software" in this Agreement). This licence is granted personally to you for use on a single computer (that is, a single Central Processing Unit).

2. This licence shall continue in force for as long as you abide by its terms and conditions. Any breach of the terms and conditions by you automatically revokes the licence without any need for notification by the copyright owner or its authorised agents.

3. As a licensee of the software you do not own what has been written nor do you own the computer program stored on the disks and it is an express condition of this licence that no right in relation to the software other than the licence set out in this Agreement is given, transferred or assigned to you.

   Ownership of the material contained in any copy of the software made by you (with authorisation or without it) remains the property of the copyright owner and unauthorised copies may also be seized in accord with the provisions of the copyright laws.

4. Copying of the software is expressly forbidden under all circumstances except one. The one exception is that you are permitted to make ONE COPY ONLY of the software on the disks for security purposes and you are encouraged to do so. This copy is referred to as the back-up copy.

5. You may transfer the software which is on the disks between computers from time to time but you agree not to use it on more than one computer at any one time and you will not transmit the contents of the disks electronically to any other. You also agree that you will not, under any circumstances, modify, adapt, translate, reverse engineer, or decompile the software or attempt any of those things.

6. Neither the licence to use the Software nor any back-up copy may be transferred to any other person without the prior written consent of WB Saunders Company Limited which consent shall not be withheld provided that the recipient agrees to be bound by the terms of licence identical to this licence. Likewise, you may not transfer, assign, lend, rent, lease, sell or otherwise dispose of the software in any packaging or upon any carrying medium other than as supplied to you by WB Saunders Company Limited. The back-up copy may not be transferred and must be destroyed if you part with possession of the software. Failure to comply with this clause will constitute a breach of this licence and may also be an infringement of copyright law.

7. It is an express condition of the licence granted to you that you disclaim any and all rights to actions or claims against WB Saunders Company Limited and/or the copyright owner with regard to any loss, injury or damage (whether to person or property and whether consequential, economic or otherwise) where any such loss, injury or damage arises directly or indirectly as a consequence (whether in whole or part):

   a) of the failure of any software contained in these disks to be fit for the purpose it has been sold whether:
      i) as a result of a defect in the software, howsoever caused; or
      ii) any defect in the carrying medium howsoever caused; and/or

   b) any other act or omission of the copyright owner or its authorised agents whatsoever,

   and you agree to indemnify WB Saunders Company Limited and the copyright owner against any and all claims, actions, suits or proceedings brought by any third party in relation to any of the above matters.

8. This agreement is to be read as subject to all local laws which are expressed to prevail over any agreement between parties to the contrary, but only to the extent that any provision in this Agreement is inconsistent with local law and no further.

9. This agreement shall be governed by the laws of the United Kingdom.